AF543016

# REMEMBER YOUR ROOTS

*Praise for*

# Remember Your Roots

"Remember Your Roots *is an incredible book that makes timeless Indigenous wisdom accessible to the descendants of any lineage so they can awaken their inner ancestral knowledge and be guided back home to their highest selves."*

— **Sahara Rose**, best-selling author and host of *Highest Self Podcast*

"Remember Your Roots *is a profound exploration of our collective lineage, intricately woven with the ancient wisdom of the Mayan people. The power of this book lies in its ability to transcend the boundaries of time and culture. It's not just about understanding Mayan wisdom; it's about rekindling a relationship with our own primal heritage, a journey toward wholeness in a fragmented world. This book is an essential read for anyone seeking to understand the interconnectedness of all life and the importance of honoring our past to navigate our future.* Remember Your Roots *is indeed a testament to the enduring power of Indigenous wisdom in shaping our collective consciousness."*

— **Ana Flores**, founder of We All Grow Latina

*"This brilliant book is a divine offering of pure love and deep ancestral wisdom. It's a generous gift to the world and one that blends ancient Indigenous wisdom with our modern times. The Mayan teachings shared throughout awaken all that is waiting to be reclaimed and remembered.* Remember Your Roots *invites us to heal in a way that our bones and blood remember—a potent journey indeed."*

— **Asha Frost**, Indigenous medicine woman and author of *You are the Medicine*

"Remember Your Roots *is an invitation to go to the depth. This book reminds you that you are more powerful than you know, and wiser than you give yourself credit for. It's a must-read for those ready to transform from the roots up."*

— **Christine Gutiérrez**, Latina therapist and author of *I Am Diosa* and *Wisdom del Alma*

# Remember Your Roots

## How to Awaken Your Ancestral Power and Live with Gratitude

(A Book Inspired by Mayan Wisdom)

By
Christine Olivia Hernandez
with Syris King-Klem

HAY HOUSE

HAY HOUSE INDIA
New Delhi • London • Sydney
Carlsbad, California • New York City

Copyright © 2024 by Christine Olivia Hernandez

**Hay House Publishers (India) Pvt Ltd**
Muskaan Complex, Plot No. 3, B-2, Vasant Kunj, New Delhi – 110070, India

Hay House LLC, P.O. Box 5100, Carlsbad, CA 92018-5100, USA
Hay House UK Ltd, 1st Floor, Crawford Corner, 91-93 Baker Street, London W1U 6QQ, UK
Hay House Australia Publishing Pty Ltd, 18/36 Ralph St., Alexandria NSW 2015, Australia

Email: contact@hayhouse.co.in
Website: www.hayhouse.co.in

*Cover design:* Mary Ann Smith
*Interior design:* Karim J. Garcia

All rights reserved. No part of this book may be reproduced by any mechanical, photographic, or electronic process, or in the form of a phonographic recording; nor may it be stored in a retrieval system, transmitted, or otherwise copied for public or private use—other than for "fair use" as brief quotations embodied in articles and reviews—without prior written permission of the publisher.

The author of this book does not dispense business advice, only offers information of a general nature to help you in your quest for business success. This book is not designed to be a definitive guide or to take the place of advice from a qualified professional, and there is no guarantee that the methods suggested in this book will be successful, owing to the risk that is involved in business of almost any kind. Thus, neither the publisher nor the author assumes liability for any losses that may be sustained by the use of the methods described in this book, and any such liability is hereby expressly disclaimed. In the event you use any of the information in this book for yourself, the author and the publisher assume no responsibility for your actions.

Names and identifying details of certain individuals have been changed to protect their privacy.

First published by Hay House India, 2025
10 9 8 7 6 5 4 3 2 1

ISBN 978-93-6611-998-4

Printed at Repro India Limited

MIX
Paper from responsible sources
FSC® C047271
FSC www.fsc.org

Hay House is committed to a sustainable future for our business, our readers and our planet. This book is made from Forest Stewardship Council® certified paper.

# CONTENTS

*We dedicate this book to my Nana Celina and Syris's mother, Elisabeth, our guardian angels, and to all our Ancestors who love us unconditionally. We also write this book for our unborn children and future generations who have yet to experience the gift of life.*

# INTRODUCTION

When I first told Syris that I wanted to write a book, I had a very different book in mind. I wanted to write a small handbook, similar to *The Four Agreements*, and it would be a simple gratitude guidebook. We'll still write that book, but as we began to channel, naturally, the creative process took on a life of its own, requiring me to reach deep within and explore all parts of myself.

As a child of an immigrant and a woman of the 21st century, I've experienced familial, relational, and systemic hardship, requiring that I work through layers of conditioning to feel genuine gratitude. It's been a confronting yet empowering process, resulting in the creation of this book. It took some time, but in the depths of my heart, I knew we were meant to write a book that offers a way to comprehensively understand ancestral healing, reconnect with nature, and find long-lasting empowerment. I thought I had done lots of work already, but to author this book meant that I was brought face-to-face with all my shadows. I was asked to explore myself deeper than ever before, allowing me to freely share what I've learned from my dynamic and magical life.

The creative process of writing and editing doesn't allow for anything to remain hidden. It brought up my deepest fears, but by using the exact practices and insights I'm sharing with you, I accessed new depths of bliss, hope, and gratitude. It's my heart's prayer that you're able to put all the pieces of yourself back together—to remember yourself—so you embody the wealth, health, and happiness that is your birthright.

## *Gratitude Is Your Birthright*

Gratitude is more than an emotion or just a temporary feeling. It is something we group together with feelings like happiness, excitement, or love, but gratitude reaches far deeper and much further than all other human emotions. I've found there are two feelings of gratitude, one for receiving and one that is an offering, a giving back, with a heartfelt openness. These are both love. It is the highest vibration as it simultaneously gives and receives. Gratitude is like the cheat code to life, for it is subtle yet powerful.

In all areas of your life, I invite you to practice feeling the subtle difference within feeling and offering gratitude without attachment to any particular thing. Flowing between the two—receiving and giving—you'll live in a state of gratitude that allows your life to unfurl in a beautiful way, giving you a divine purpose. When we learn to live gratefully, we live in peace and in balance with all things, remembering that we are a part of the whole. Living with a sense of connection, purpose, and hope, we will do our part to make the world a better place.

Gratitude is a staple attribute of Indigenous cultures across the planet. From the Aboriginals in Australia to the Celts in Europe, from the Shipibo in South America to the Kanaka Maoli in Hawaii, from diverse Indigenous peoples in North America to the Maya in Mesoamerica, and so many others, gratitude and living in reciprocity is a defining aspect of daily life. My Mayan elders and guides practice giving thanks to everything daily: for being alive, the things that sustain life, our comforts, the elements, animals, the sun, stars, trees, their breath, and so forth. This allows them to appreciate life and honor the Spirit within all things. Reciprocity is the act of being reverent for what we are given, and giving our gratitude is the ultimate way to be fair, equitable, and in harmony.

Tata Izaias, a Mayan spiritual guide and friend, shared with me, "After we have eaten a meal, we say, 'Maltyox Chra Qa Way' (thank you for our food), and we answer as 'Ajaw Xyioh' (the Spirit provided)." Gratitude is shared from our hearts, not just empty words, in order to acknowledge the Spirit within everything. Another powerful phrase he shared is Oxlajuj Maltyoxil, which means "13 times thank you." In Mayan traditions, oxlajuj, or "13," represents completeness, and *maltyox* translates to "thank you." Therefore, Oxlajuj Maltyoxil is a way of giving gratitude to everything and everyone, even for the things that aren't named or aren't remembered.

I'm blessed to have found a home in Totonicapán, spending time with my teachers Nana Lu, Nana Maria, and Tata Tino, the K'iche' Maya lineage with whom, at the time of publishing this book, I am being initiated as an Aj Q'ij, also known as a Mayan Day Keeper or spiritual guide. While there, I've witnessed the authentic lives of the Maya, untouched by tourism in Guatemala. They express gratitude before meals and after eating; they personally thank each individual present. Sharing their homes and participating in their ceremonies is incredibly heartwarming and has brought much clarity to my life. It revealed how they live in a genuine state of gratitude, leading seemingly simple lives, but filled with richness, community, purpose, and connection.

## *The Flow of the Book*

This book offers you a transformation out of fear and into bliss, with gratitude as a defining practice to help you make this shift. The 13 chapters are written and structured in a specific order to support you knowing and healing all aspects of yourself.

We begin with your physical body, for all true healing happens by beginning with the body. Your body is your starting point, your anchor, and your vessel from which you have a human experience. Understanding, connecting with, and opening up to the wisdom of your body begins what will be a beautiful journey of remembrance and reclamation.

We then move into the mind, helping you to create a supportive mental environment and continuing to strengthen your foundation. Next, we outline the mystery that is your soul, discovering the unique imprint that makes you, *you*. Rippling out, we show how to create safe, vulnerable, and loving relationships with others now that you've begun accessing the innate wisdom and power of your body, mind, and soul. We then move into showing how your Ancestors are essential parts of who you are, extensions of your relationships, and that your lineage wants you to live a beautiful, abundant life. There are also generational patterns that we must tend to so we don't repeat unhealthy cycles.

Thankfully, you are infinitely supported on this path! To open you up to the abundance that life has for you, in the next chapter we offer how plants, animals, and the natural world are here so you can create a life filled with health, vitality, and gratitude. Then, the following four chapters dive into the four elements of earth, fire, water, and air, each providing often-forgotten wisdom that will further open your heart and mind. These elements are your most ancient Ancestors, and they have much to teach you about yourself.

The next chapter speaks to the power, potency, and need for ceremony. Life itself is a ceremony, yet many have forgotten how to celebrate or set aside time to honor how sacred our lives truly are. This chapter reminds you how to honor both the light and the dark, and how through celebration, prayer, and gratitude, you'll discover true fulfillment. Next, we speak to magic, and through healing our inner child, we can tap into that which is seen and unseen to create the life of our dreams. To conclude, we show how most live in a search to love or be loved. This is usually a pure-hearted desire, yet it can often leave us unfulfilled. Therefore, we show that living in a state of gratitude is the best way to create a life of bliss.

### *The Heart of This Book*

The wisdom within this book is a blend between the traditional teachings of my Mayan lineage and my learned experience as someone who's devoted my entire life to awakening, healing, and being in a personal relationship with the Divine. It is through both inheritance, devotion, and training that I've reclaimed my truth as a medicine woman, a guide, and a voice standing in my power for myself and for my Ancestors who could not.

This book is inspired by my Mayan lineage's wisdom, teachings, and cosmovision, which is complex and dynamic. Since most teachings have been burned or lost, some traditions maintain a sense of exclusivity. Most teachings that remain have metaphorical or figurative interpretations. The few texts that weren't burned by Spanish priests during colonization mostly speak about origin myths and don't have direct information about culture, ceremony, and practices. Oral traditions, safeguarded by wisdom keepers, blend with knowledge from archaeological discoveries. Together, with the profound experiences from visions and traditional rites of passage, we can piece together a fuller picture of our history.

Those who study Mayan wisdom are working with limited information, yet it is obvious that the power and scope of Mayan wisdom is beyond what most anyone can imagine. Learning from the wisdom keepers of ancient traditions can and will change your life. When we learn from Indigenous teachings, your heart's intention is most important. We must learn to appreciate, not appropriate, the sacred practices of all Indigenous teachings. Regardless of descent, we must respect and honor their medicine, but remember, the ultimate authority is how God, Creator, the unnamable one that goes by a thousand names, moves through you. Truth is not limited to words in a book or those spoken by an elder, guide, or priest. We do this work to remember our roots not only for ourselves, but for the greatest good of all.

When we remember our roots, we remember our truth, finding that we are connected to the wisdom of the trees, the light of stars, all parts of nature, the elements, and to life itself. We find that we belong to so much more than previously realized and that we are all kin. In this way, we will live in right relationship and find boundless gratitude for all things. It is my honor to bridge these ancient teachings to the modern day so that you can also connect to your roots and live a life of greater wholeness, for no matter your specific descent, we are all connected.

Each of us has a unique lineage, yet if we trace our roots back, we find that we share wise Ancestors who lived in harmony. I am referring to our most ancient Ancestors, not the ones who lived through, experienced, or participated in various forms of colonization. The wisdom of the wise and ancient ways is in your blood, and as human beings, we are all stewards of the Earth. These Ancestors were thankful for all things and honored the Great Mystery of this life. It's essential we honor each culture's uniqueness, yet ultimately, we are all connected, each a part of the Divine and a unique expression of a shared Oneness. It is time to remember these wise ways of the past and release harmful practices that have become normalized within our current societal structures.

### *About Us*

I am a second-generation immigrant, born and raised in and around Riverside, California. My paternal lineage is of Mayan and mixed descent from Guatemala, and my maternal lineage is of Mexican and American descent. I have descended from Indigenous Ancestors who did not have fair or equitable opportunities to share their voices, or be connected to their truth, magic, and purpose. Therefore, it is my honor and responsibility to use my voice to share the magic of my lineage. I do this for myself, for my Ancestors who could not, and the many generations who will come after me.

It's taken time to re-Indigenize my mind, but by honoring my Indigenous heritage as well as the influences of colonization in my ancestry, I can live in greater wholeness. We cannot change who we are or where we come from, nor should we try. I am proud of my mixed blood with all its wisdom as well as the shortcomings of my lineage. All of us descend from both victim and perpetrator. Through this process of remembering my roots, I've gathered information, skills, and techniques, coming to fully understand how I am made of both the light and the dark. I am made of dirt and stars. I am part human, part wild woman. I have fire in my heart, water in my blood, earth as my body, and the wind as my breath. And you, my kin, do too.

Every human holds an ancient history within our blood. Since I am a descendant of mixed race and ancestry, I have much to learn from the past. I can do better than my Ancestors that caused harm, and I can restore the beauty of those who were wise in their ways. What resonates with me can stay, and what does not can end with me. If I can become the change maker, the cycle breaker, and the liberator of my bloodline by owning my life story, then so can you.

My husband and co-author, Syris, was instrumental in supporting me writing, editing, and getting this book published. He is an ally to marginalized communities, and while he has a vastly different background than me, he's experienced things within his life that have given him a unique depth. He is an Air Force veteran, and he supports many authors as a cross-genre book writer and editor. He's also a screenwriter and actor, having devoted his life to the mastery of storytelling, knowing that through the words we use and the stories we tell, we can shift, determine, and recreate reality.

We met in Guatemala in February 2020, and just days after meeting, lockdowns required that we stay in the country, resulting in us living together for over four months! Since then, he's been my greatest ally, creative collaborator, and the loving partner I dreamed of, and we've grown through it all. This book wouldn't exist without his creative direction, giving me the structure I needed to write *this*, the book I wish I had throughout my journey.

Also, this book is proof that the most powerful creations are done as collaborations, showing what can be made when peoples of vastly different lineages come together with tenderness, curiosity, and a heart of service. For that, and for him, I am eternally grateful.

## *We Root and Rise Together*

We find ourselves in a time where the world is rapidly changing, yet the wisdom within this book is timeless. At this present time, we are being asked to do more than simply continue traditions and cultures. We are being asked to integrate the teachings of the wise Ancestors and bridge ancient wisdom to modern practical use and understanding. We are being called to do the work to heal so that together, we may live with greater harmony. By healing past traumas and embodying gratitude for all to see, we can hold up a light in the darkness, becoming the leaders of our lineage as humanity makes a massive shift into a new paradigm.

There is a mass awakening happening across the planet, but many people are heavily programmed, keeping them disconnected, fearful, and stuck in ways that do not resonate any longer. It can seem easier to harden ourselves to the world after we've been bruised and beaten, but what is truly powerful is to remain openhearted. It takes practice, but it is our responsibility to alchemize our pain into our purpose. Through that process, we learn how to be more loving and compassionate. When we are truly grateful for all things, not just saying we are, but after truly putting in the work, we start to see things differently. We become empowered. We become responsible for our thoughts, actions, and decisions. We learn how to do and be and live better. We cannot be truly grateful and condone hurtful behaviors. Only with a grateful heart can we send ripples of love, bliss, and peace out into the world.

Many people have heard about having a gratitude journal, but just writing or speaking on gratitude doesn't make a big enough impact. So I offer Embodiment Practices at the end of each chapter, and some more simple ones scattered throughout, to create long-lasting effects and a sustained sense of gratitude. When we feel grateful in our body, it makes it real. At first, we may need to use our imagination to make it real, but the more we practice, the more we will start to truly feel it.

Repetition is the key to making something second nature, yet you may find it hard to be grateful at first. Some of the Embodiment Practices may not fully resonate, but I recommend that you do your best to experience them fully. They may seem odd, simple, or whimsical. Regardless, allow yourself to feel whatever you feel, but still do them. Trust me; there is an ancient intelligence behind each one.

We must be persistent—and consistent—to live a life of gratitude. Our minds have been hardwired for negativity, so it's essential to be compassionate with yourself. Know that you possess all the power you need to create a new reality. The more you make gratitude a habit in your daily life, the more grateful you will feel, and the more you will find things to be grateful for. It's a beautiful and empowering way to live.

Remembering your roots is the starting point for this transformative journey. As we root and rise together, we not only empower ourselves but also create a ripple effect that reaches those around us. This collective rooting and rising amplifies the gratitude you can give and receive, building a life based on thankfulness and reciprocity.

By acknowledging where you come from and recognizing the power of your interconnectedness, you pave the way for a more grateful, balanced, and empathetic society. It all starts with remembering your roots and choosing to rise in gratitude. This is how you will bear rich fruit for yourself, your loved ones, and all those who will come after you.

CHAPTER 1:

# In Your Body Is a Good Place to Be

*"In your body is a good place to be."*

— Beatrix Ost

For over 3,000 years, my ancient Mayan and Mexica* Ancestors built temples, pyramids, and sacred sites all over Mesoamerica. They built these sites to protect life-giving springs of water, aligned them with the stars above, and to honor all aspects of life, from birth to death, seasons and cycles, and the elements. People native to the Americas were in right relationship with the lands they lived on and the natural world that supported every aspect of their life. These ancient Ancestors embodied the understanding that life is sacred, and all things are connected.

In the present day, we have the incredible gift of having access to both ancient wisdom teachings and modern medicine. We may romanticize past eras, but we have

*Pronounced Meh-shee-ka, Mexica is the original Nahuatl name for the people in Mexico who are known in the Western world as Azteca or Aztecs. The term *Aztec* was given to them after colonization, used to collectively describe Nahuatl-speaking peoples in the region of central Mexico in the post-classic period, but it was not a term used by the Mexica to describe themselves.

distracted ourselves from simple things that were once considered holy. Humanity's scientific ability to look closer into the microcosm of our own body and simultaneously look further into the macrocosm of the furthest reaches of the Universe has captivated our attention. But with how many inputs we have and seemingly endless streams of information, many people, just like I did, lose sight of and completely forget how and why all things are interconnected.

It was the role of our ancient Ancestors to build these sacred sites with various intentions to remind us of who we are and what is most essential. Now it's our responsibility to recognize that our physical body is a temple that is the home to an eternal, undying spirit. You are the creation of those who survived earthquakes, famine, sickness, and violence. Your existence itself is a miracle, one that has defied all odds to give you the breath in your lungs, a spark in your heart, life in your blood, and movement in your bones. Your body is the ultimate sacred site: a temple to honor all things past and present and an altar made up of sacred waters, hummingbird feathers, primordial elements, living organisms, and ancient stardust.

The health of your body is a reflection of how intentional you are. How deeply you are connected to your body determines how much bliss and fulfillment you will be able to access, for it is through the body that we experience life. Understanding yourself and coming into right relationship with your body is the essential starting point.

## *Beginning to Feel It All*

For the majority of my remembered life, I was completely lost and disconnected from my body, unwilling to let myself feel too deeply. I couldn't or didn't want to acknowledge the pain, grief, and disappointment I carried. As can be common for someone born into the family dynamics, society, and fragmented culture I received as the child of a Guatemalan immigrant and second-generation Mexican American, I armored my heart for as long as I could. Eventually, I normalized being completely closed off. If I stayed armored and didn't let people into my heart, I thought they couldn't hurt me deeply. Another protective mechanism I used was to physically disassociate. If I felt too vulnerable, I'd check out so that I didn't feel the full effects of heartache. However, a core knot was being tied at the deepest roots of my personal identity, defining my beliefs and how I began to relate with everything in my life, and the fabric of life itself.

Dissociation is a learned behavior that can result from childhood neglect, abandonment, or abuse. If no one is there to stand up for us or support us as children, we dissociate from the pain to provide a short-term escape. If we shut ourselves off to feeling pain in the short-term, we will become too numb to deeply feel pleasure, bliss, or gratitude. If you're feeling a painful feeling, emotion, or body sensation, or if you're feeling numb, the most common next step people take is to feel bad about feeling bad. This loop of self-imposed shame is also a learned behavior that keeps millions of people believing they are depressed, sick, and that there is something "wrong" with them.

I get it; it can be scary to recognize that we're in pain. Often, it seems so much easier to just numb out. If you're like me, then admitting you're in pain just makes the source of that pain real, and so we cling to the feeling that life shouldn't be so damn hard. We hope everyone isn't just going to hurt us if we open our heart, and maybe if we pretend long enough that our pain isn't real, someone or something else will come along and make it better.

The core belief that the world was fundamentally an unsafe place was firmly etched into my belief system. Deep within my subconscious, a protective part of me felt safe holding on to my distrust because if shit hit the fan, then that part of me would be there for me. That part would say something like, "I told you this would happen. See, that is why I was here with this wall to protect you from any further heartbreak." When disconnected to the wisdom of your body, and being controlled by your mind, you'll always find evidence for what you choose to believe. If the mind is like wind, your body is like rock—the winds can whip you all around or a rock can crush you with its weight. But in time, you will learn how to stay grounded in your body, able to listen to your innate wisdom even when the winds of the mind whip within.

Holding on to self-protective mechanisms, I thought I could predict the outcomes in life, not realizing that my "predicting" was actually creating situations that only deepened a fear-based view of life. I thought I was effectively controlling my reactions by not getting too vulnerable, so I seemed to feel all right in the end. But this way of experiencing things didn't serve the highest vision for my life, nor does it serve yours. When someone reflected to me that I still had walls up and was prepared for emotional defense, it took time, and Embodiment Practices I will share at the end of each chapter, to soften and surrender my need for control.

As a child, since I didn't have anyone to show me how to not take other people's frustrations, anger, or abuse personally, a part of me believed that what they were saying was true. I began to believe the lie that something was wrong with me. As an adult, I had to give myself what I needed to unlearn those stories and rediscover my true identity. When I'd get triggered, it was because something was hitting a wounded place still within me. Since I learned to take on other people's truth, whenever I felt bad, unworthy, or not good enough, that was the only thing that seemed to be real.

You must recognize that you are not wrong or bad for what you feel because there's always a deeper truth at play. Instead of dissociating and numbing out, you can realize it's okay for it to be hard to actually be in your body. At first, it is challenging to sit with difficult feelings because an aspect of ourselves feels like they're real. Yet, when we give space to feel all feelings, those feelings inevitably dissipate, and a sense of a deeper truth moves into place. It takes only practice and the commitment to be the best version of yourself.

Ultimately, you are the witness of the drama that unfolds, past and present, but that doesn't define you. The true you is not only the wounded parts, the one who numbs out, or the one who feels like you'll never be "enough." With so many aspects to the self, it's important to not prefer one version over another, but rather feel what you feel, moment to moment, and allow the unfolding challenges of your life to be invitations to stop responding out of fear and come into deeper embodiments of gratitude.

### *The Three Phases*

Something I use to help me identify how deeply embodied I am at any given time and in any given situation are the three phases that manifest in all aspects of life. For example: when I want to feel connected, safe, or anything else that seems better than what I am feeling, I am in Phase One. It's unconsciously living our lives defined by a sense of need, whether we actually allow ourselves to realize it or not. Living predominantly in Phase One keeps us on the surface, meaning we're never deeply rooted and we resist diving into why we feel, experience, and believe what we do. While there is nothing wrong with wanting to feel better, our initial desires are usually not coming from an embodied place. That's where Phase Two comes in and plays its role perfectly.

As it relates to being present in your body, Phase Two is living hardened and seemingly disconnected from everything. This happens by being repeatedly hurt, disappointed, or left unfulfilled. It's making the agreement with ourself that life is too much to deal with and that's just the way things are. Living with this sense of separation, I drank heavily, religiously kept things surface in all my relationships, and found escape in food, entertainment, social media, boyfriends, my work, and so on. When you're dissociated from what life is showing you or wishing things were different, better, or easier, then you're not allowing yourself to grow. Remember, armoring comes from needing to protect yourself, and numbness is what blocks you from experiencing the bliss that is your birthright. In this chapter, and throughout the entire book, I'm going to show you how and why to move through Phases One and Two. We'll access the essential information both stages are trying to show you so that you may ultimately create a life by your own design.

Living in Phase Three is not the utopian fulfillment to soothe your suffering, but here magic *is* real, and miracles *do* happen. It's not separate from Phases One and Two, but instead, deeply connected to them. When in Phase Three and you feel like life is hard or something hurtful happens, you don't shift your attention outside of yourself and numb out, you first look within. Then, you will set strong boundaries to ensure your continued embodiment of bliss, knowing you deserve to live a magical life. By keeping your focus on being present in your body, the world you create for yourself will become a place where you are supported and completely safe.

Difficult past experiences can make us remain in a fight, flight, freeze, or fawn trauma response which keeps us in Phases One or Two. Only after allowing yourself the time to fully process past and present experiences can you learn that your true, inner self remains safe, even during challenging times, without automatically resorting to defending, appeasing, or disassociating when faced with external threats. Regardless of circumstance, presence whispers, "Give me a chance." When you listen to that whisper, you'll not feel bad for feeling bad, but instead ask, "Okay, I'm listening. What do you have to show me?"

In Phase Three, there are no skipping steps of feeling. You have to feel it to heal it. You are the only one who is going to save you, and you're the only person you can change. The versions of you that other people have are theirs. How people treat you actually has nothing to do with you, but no one can know you like you know you. Be gentle with yourself, feel your feelings, hold yourself accountable when you try to reach outside of yourself, listen to what your life is trying to teach you, speak your truth with love, and do your best to be present in your body throughout it all. Doing this, you can't help but begin to untie all the knots that keep you bound up and find the golden thread of gratitude that will weave your entire life into wholeness.

## *Knowing vs. Gnosis*

Familial, collective, and systemic abuse, coupled with colonization and improper uses of patriarchy, have kept generation after generation armored, but thankfully, we do not have to carry on in these ways. By recognizing the importance of being present in our body, and that it's not something to just think but practice, we can acknowledge that underneath it all we feel things and we can do something about them. Every single person has the ability and responsibility to explore their pain and find resolution for the things others have done to hurt them, as well as how they've hurt themselves or others as a result.

Pain is information from the past or present that we have yet to find a place for. In a world where there's a pill for every symptom of our deep-rooted knots, this is the least prescribed and the hardest pill to swallow, but it takes time, patience, practice, and healthy internal and external environments to find deep healing. Only when we give ourselves what we truly need, can we find the strength, confidence, and safety to feel our feelings, to say the things out loud that we've kept inside, and stop dissociating from our body. Then we can find and weave gratitude into our life, and truly love being in our body in all ways, always. This may take time, so be easy on yourself, but the positive impacts are instant.

Even now, I still find myself making excuses or having expectations that since I "know" these things, I must be healthy, empowered, and embodied, right? Kind of, but there's a difference between knowing something in your head and knowing it in your body. The word *knowledge* comes from the Greek word *gnosis*, which means to know something deeply, far beyond just the facts.

Gnosis can also be understood through the phases we just covered. Phase One is knowing something like, "I want to be healthier, so I should have a daily fitness routine." After overcoming the resistance of that phase, you enter into Phase Two. Then, you're likely to feel like you're never going to be "fit enough" or like you'll never reach your goals, so you make excuses to not work out. Phase Two is defined by a sense of separation, and in this example, feeling separate from where you are and where you want to be. After overcoming that sense of separation, in Phase Three, you once again "know" that it's healthy to have a daily fitness routine, but now that you've gone through Phase Two and chosen to do the work to achieve your goals, you develop a deep gnosis in your body that you are healthy, happy, and whole. And anytime you feel afraid to begin the next stage of your growth (Phase One) or like you'll never get there no matter what you do (Phase Two), you're able to quickly recognize this within yourself. Placing your attention and intention on taking action instead of reacting, you will experience the embodied wisdom of Phase Three.

Developing your ability to feel, sense, and connect with your feelings, emotions, and bodily sensations throughout each phase is your quickest way to find gratitude. It takes time, practice, and patience, for at first, gratitude is a subtle thread, but once you do, its golden radiance will illuminate your life, filling it with beauty, pleasure, and bliss like you've never known. This took me years to learn, and every new day, and really each moment, is another opportunity to be present in my body and grateful for the miracle it is to be alive.

### *Open, Feel, and Heal*

I know I'm not alone in the fact that I have experienced many traumas in my past. Like millions of children, I was abandoned by my father when I was an infant and raised by a young, single mother. She did the best she could, yet sometimes, she left me feeling unsafe and neglected. I experienced and witnessed physical, emotional, mental, and verbal abuse in most of my households. Yelling, name calling, threatening, beatings with a belt, and hair pulling weren't unusual occurrences. I was deeply troubled, and there were many reasons why I felt unsafe being in my body and just living in the world. It's taken a lot of time, a lot of patience, and countless hours of deep self-help work, but now I can claim in complete gratitude that every experience has gotten me to where I am now.

Like my beloved friend Beatrix often says, "In my body is a good place to be." To be able to say this with complete truth, you can't skip any steps. Just because you know about the phases that play out in any given situation, it doesn't serve you to bypass what you're really feeling in Phase Two or ignore the fear of Phase One. To just say, "I'm so grateful," is a trap that will block you from experiencing the heights of joy, pleasure, and gratitude that you deserve to feel every single day. You deserve to feel enraptured with life by infusing your body, mind, and soul with authentic, embodied gratitude. This is a lifelong process of healing and remembering our truth. Go as slow as you need to while you peel back layers of grief, getting to the deepest roots of who you are.

Just like the sacred sites ancient peoples made to preserve information and remind us of who we are, our body stores memory within its tissue. The depth of bliss we feel is proportionate to overcoming what holds us back.

It's hard for empowering beliefs to take root when we are filled with unprocessed trauma, subconscious limiting beliefs, and old habits. To truly heal, we need to address these issues at their roots so that our soils will be fertile for our evolution. Like peeling an onion, we heal layer by layer. This means we do not turn away from feeling pain, anger, or sorrow because it's showing us a deeper layer of something we need to recognize. We must shake free from the shackles our body has been in to feel safe and welcome in more gratitude for everything our life is showing us. By doing so, we open ourselves up to greater joy and pleasure.

I am on this healing journey with you. When triggers happen, I am learning to not take someone else, myself, or the situation personally. It takes time to shift into gratitude, but I know that there's something I need on the other side of feeling the pain associated with wounds. Whether I have words for the feelings or not, I do my best to keep my walls down, take my armor off, and stay present in my body. Even though it can be hard, I try not to shame myself for not being fully healed and perfect. I remember that my beloved, business partners, or family members are ultimately my teammates and do not blame them for triggering me or hurting me, but seek out resolution after I've had time to feel safety and come into a regulated state. I no longer numb or disassociate, but instead I open, I feel, and I heal.

### *The Intelligence Within*

Because of colonization and the continued embrace of Catholicism, almost all Indigenous Mayan wisdom teachings have been lost. Also, the codices that survived being burned by Spanish Catholic priests have been translated from the native language to Spanish and now English. There are also oral teachings, but those are open to interpretation, and sometimes even manipulation. For over the last 500 years, few have devoted their lives to understanding the original essence of Mayan wisdom without the dogma and hierarchy that has gripped nearly all aspects of modern culture. This is why to actually understand the incredibly useful, life-changing, and profound wisdom of the Maya, one must be able to feel in their own body what resonates and what does not. A student of these teachings must be coming to learn with a pure heart. This doesn't mean they must be perfect already, nor should they give their power away to a specific teacher or tradition. All you need is a desire to deepen your embodiment and come with a grateful heart. The more you explore, the more these teachings will bring you into deep remembrance and clear gnosis of what the ancient Maya did their best to preserve for us today.

Sadly, most modern Maya don't realize that the fast food, Catholic/Evangelical teachings, and alcoholism that have consumed thousands of husbands and fathers are direct impacts of colonization. I know that my Mayan Ancestors, just like your most ancient Ancestors, lived far differently before there were any of these destructive influences. When we tap into the intelligence of our own bodies, feel our loving and wise Ancestors supporting us, and embrace our connection to the natural world, we can learn and remember far more than relying on elders who may or may not be free from the enduring impacts of toxic forms of patriarchy. For example, the Mayan way of becoming a spiritual guide does not only happen by being anointed by another person through a hierarchy. They may receive their gifts or power from the unseen realms, through dreams, through illness, or the Sign they are born with.

So much of translated Mayan wisdom speaks to connecting with the outer world, the wisdom of the planet, and the Cosmos. This is a beautiful and important element of feeling wholeness, but what I found missing in most elders is a deep connection to their own bodies. While it is highly beneficial and critical to learn from elders, they are also imperfect humans. We must remember to not put anyone on a pedestal or take away a teacher's or mentor's humanity just because it seems like they know more than we do. Everyone is doing their best, yet everyone is shaped by their unique experiences and has their own biases. All of us have been impacted by colonization and negative forms of patriarchy, whether we are aware of it or not.

There is an innate wisdom within our DNA that holds the potential for personal empowerment and growth. However, it takes effort and conscious work to activate and awaken your inner power. By living from this empowered place, you will form better relationships while also engaging intentionally with the external world. It's important to balance these internal sources of wisdom with external knowledge and find harmony with both. This is why it is essential to tap into the divine feminine within. By connecting with the divine feminine, you'll cultivate qualities like intuition, empathy, and emotional intelligence, which are often undervalued or dismissed in current systems. Doing so will create healthier relationships to ourselves, our mentors, and the world around us.

In one instance, I did a weeklong womb healing training, learning how to activate the heart of the stomach from the world-renowned Mayan midwife Doña Dominga and my sister-friend Mariu. While there, I learned how our wombs hold on to things that have affected them in the past. Memory gets stored in the body, and challenging experiences can leave lasting effects with our monthly cycles, reproduction, and hormonal balance if we do not tend to our womb. When it comes to physical effects like yeast infections, bladder infections, or bacterial infections, we can heal these imbalances with herbs and our diet. If our pelvis is misaligned or our womb holds tension, we can move the heart of the stomach back into place and support realignment with direct touch.

During the opening ceremony for our teachings, we drank Mayan ceremonial cacao to open our hearts and activate our wombs. I will never forget how Mariu shared with the group that while she had learned so much from our elder, Doña Dominga, Mariu had taught Doña that by beginning with body massage, they could relax the women before doing the deep work. The "work" to move things into alignment is emotionally taxing, is not physically subtle or gentle, and can sometimes cause people to disassociate from their body. However, by beginning the session with gentleness, the impact was even more substantial, and we were able to breathe into and relax through the necessary discomfort.

The Maya have many guardians of their culture and most work toward sharing the wisdom of the Ancestors in order to create a brighter future for all. However, we must not rely on anyone or anything for our healing or to feel safe and supported. When we remember our inner wisdom and remain the students of all that life has to teach us, we blossom into our full expression of who we're destined to be. Your lineage, your past life experiences, your dietary decisions, and how balanced you are in your health all are access points for you to remember you are whole and holy, emanations of magic, and the embodiment of, and the perfect reflection of, the divine Creator. All parts of life hold wisdom and medicine for us, but ultimately, you are the medicine. May you remember to remain a student with a grateful and humble heart while simultaneously knowing that the deepest wisdom available to you is within your own body.

### *Embodiment Practice: Holding Yourself*

This is a self-love practice that I recommend doing daily or whenever you're feeling overwhelmed, numb, or amid anything that tends to take you out of your body. You deserve to feel loved, and loving yourself first is key to a happy, healthy, and harmonious life. If you skip the step of practicing self-love, you will be bypassing an essential element of healing. We cannot be loving to others if we do not first feel loved within ourselves. This is also a practice to use when you are feeling triggered. Hold yourself as soon as you feel any sense of discomfort. Feeling held will remind you that you are okay, you are safe, and you are always held and supported.

To begin, take a look around the room you are in and notice where you are. Notice if you feel safe or uncomfortable in this space. See the walls, the floors, the furniture, and take note of how it feels to sit where you are sitting. Feel the cushion beneath you and feel from the top of your head to the soles of your feet. When you can feel yourself arriving and present in the body, close your eyes and take a few deep breaths to fully feel your body relax. With every breath, notice your body softening.

Start to bring your arms around you in an embrace. Squeeze your arms, moving your hands up and down your arms, hugging yourself gently. Stay in this embrace for a few minutes, simply breathing and being aware of the sensation of feeling yourself being held by yourself. Ask yourself how it feels to be giving and receiving your own love and care.

When you're ready, allow your hands to move back down your arms and across your legs. Slowly rub your belly, making circles clockwise with the gentle weight of your palm for a minute or so. Those with a womb, pause to gently send love to your womb. Next, massage your legs and feet. Bring your hands up to your shoulders and massage your shoulders. Relax into receiving your own gentle loving touch. Remember you deserve to feel good, and you deserve your own love. Lastly, bring your hands to your head and finish the massage by rubbing your temples and head in a nurturing way. When you feel complete, bring your hands to prayer in front of your heart. Gently open your eyes, acknowledging where you are in space and time, expressing gratitude for all *you've* just felt, remembered, and reconnected to.

CHAPTER 2:

# Your Mind Is a Garden

*"You don't become what you want; you become what you believe."*

— Oprah Winfrey

To cultivate a garden is no small task—there are pests, diseases, hungry critters, and all kinds of environmental challenges that can harm what you're growing. Our mind is like a garden, and for it to flourish, we must constantly tend to it. If it's neglected, it will become overgrown and fruitless from intrusive thoughts, mental storms, and unstable conditions. If you perceive things that cause pain as a threat, you'll likely become reactive and feel like other people, or your own mind, is an enemy. When your mind is an ally, you'll have the confidence to respond well to things that challenge you.

You also must keep your mind-garden healthy by clearing yourself from intrusive thoughts as if you're pulling out unwanted weeds. If you want to take a shortcut, you can use pesticide and weed killer, but if you do so, you're infusing your precious soil with toxic chemicals. Many people have become dependent on quick results, like some fast-acting prescriptions for anxiety, depression, and other psychological imbalances, just like many gardeners use Roundup for pests and weeds.

Note: In Chapter 6, we'll dive deep into how these "weeds" are actually essential medicines that have been used for thousands of years for holistic healing; in this chapter, I'll show you how intrusive, "negative" thoughts actually hold essential information that we must learn to honor.

While I have personally used pharmaceutical prescriptions in the past to support mental distress—and understand that in some cases, these medications can be lifesaving and enhancing—I came to realize that for me personally, the compounding negative impacts for short-term benefits weren't worth it. Since your mind is like fertile soil, what you take in via medicine, food, entertainment, and social media is what determines the quality of life you're able to experience.

Amid being so intent on clearing your mind-garden from small, pesky things, if you get tunnel vision on a single problem, you may forget to look up and check the weather. The sun could scorch your plants if you don't cover them, or a hurricane could come along and destroy everything you've cultivated. I know how overwhelming it is to try and manage small troubles in your daily life but also have to watch out for things that can come along and mentally blow us away. Unhealthy relationships, toxic work environments, intense global events, and other big-picture problems can seemingly uproot us, leaving us devastated and mentally drained. Therefore, you must continually determine for yourself if certain relationships and environments are fueling you into a grateful life or grinding down your spirit.

For example, activism, social justice, and climate change awareness are all essential topics that deserve your attention; however, you must first tend to your own well-being before trying to make any real change in the world. If you try to change something for the better—like a difficult relationship dynamic—but you're feeling frazzled, what you create won't be of the highest quality. A thriving garden isn't built in a day. Juicy fruits and nourishing veggies don't sprout overnight. The rains will come, and the winds will blow. But through it all, by keeping things simple, utilizing the practices in this book, and prioritizing a healthy mental state, you will create an abundant, bustling garden with goodness to share with many.

To have a healthy mind-garden, you also must know in which season to plant, when to harvest, and when to take a break. In this way, going to therapy, seeking out new healing methods, or exploring deeper layers of your mental health is best done in seasons and cycles. Since healing is like peeling an onion, with every layer you peel back, you find more of the same thing, but with added complexities. The deeper you go, the closer you get to the source. That's why there is no rush to figure it all out, because no matter where you look, you're going to find the same things appearing in different forms.

It's critical to take breaks, prioritize periods of deep rest, and integrate what you are experiencing just like gardens do during the peak of summer or the coldest part of winter. It's in these resting seasons that what you've previously grown, harvested, and stored will sustain you. However, if you rush the process, you'll feel powerless, incapable, and will solely rely on other people to feel nourished. If you feel that other people have it better than you, like it's too hard to have good mental health, or you rely on other people to feel safe, these are signals to slow down, align with your own cycles (I share how to do this in Chapter 7), and listen to your inner guidance.

### *You Are What You Eat*

This mind-garden analogy goes a few steps deeper because mental health and the quality of food you eat go hand in hand. Eating organic, non-processed food will support you in having a healthy gut microbiome, make new connections in your brain, and regulate your nervous system. You'll have more energy and focus, and who knows what opportunities you will be able to recognize and act upon by giving yourself all the essential minerals, fats, proteins, and vitamins you need to not only survive, but thrive!

I know how hard it is to eat well. Born into a low-income, Westernized family, I was raised eating highly processed foods. I was nutrient deficient for most of my life, and I used to have major stomach issues growing up. After several doctors' visits around the age of 18, I found out I had IBS, acid reflux, and lactose intolerance. That led me to want to learn more about nutrition so that I could stop eating the foods that were causing me pain. Little by little I began to educate myself, prioritize my health, and make changes in my diet.

When I learned of my stomach issues, my go-to meal was pizza with ranch, and a salad drenched in extra ranch. It (seemed to be) affordable, delicious, and because I had a salad, I thought it was good for me. Everyone is so different, so it's not just about applying what is working for someone else; it's about seeing what feels good for you after learning what isn't working. I went from eating pizzas to grocery store sushi, which was also difficult to process, especially since I didn't chew my food long enough. I'd also eat frozen foods and think that was healthy because the box said so. I didn't know what organic really was till my mid-20s, let alone regenerative.

I could write a whole book on the importance of food, but what I will suggest is to start slowly. Make incremental changes. You don't need to throw everything out and replace your food overnight. Go slow. Buy organic foods as much as you can. Drink clean water. Shop at farmers markets and local co-ops. Eat slowly, be present with your food, and chew your food until it's mush. Drink less with your meals. Let yourself digest for at least 5 to 10 minutes before you hop up to go do the next thing. It took me time to get it right, and it wasn't until I was in my late 20s that I learned the critical importance of eating organic produce, grass-fed meats, wild-caught fish, and more fruits and veggies. It was a hard loop to get out of, especially when healthy foods seemed to be so much more expensive, require more work to prepare, and did not taste as good. However, with effort, it can be done.

Eating well does not need to be more expensive or complicated; it can be fairly simple and affordable. People tend to eat much more meat in the Western World, yet they aren't living as long as people in Nicoya, Costa Rica, who eat less meat and eat a diet consisting of maize (corn), squash, and beans otherwise known as "the Three Sisters," which I discuss in the next section of this chapter. Nicoya is considered a Blue Zone. A "Blue Zone" is a region where people are observed to live longer, healthier lives, often reaching ages well beyond the global average. Not only that, but these Native people are also reportedly 10 years younger biologically. This Blue Zone is diminishing because the youth are not following the Ancestral diets but rather turning to fast food, which is sadly becoming more popular and accessible in their region.

At first, changing dietary habits can be challenging. Your taste buds might need time to adjust. But, once they do, you'll find that you no longer crave foods that ultimately give you discomfort or have little nutritional value. Over time, you will find yourself wanting less sodium, sugar, and processed junk foods. This isn't just about developing discipline; it's about addressing underlying nutritional needs. Often, our cravings arise because our minds are used to certain routines. Other times, and more importantly, our bodies are in dire need of essential nutrients, which can also create cravings. When we provide our bodies with the right nourishment, intense cravings that come from our mind or body will diminish.

Hippocrates, the "Father of Western Medicine," is widely known to have said, "Let food be thy medicine." Sadly, Western medicine and our society at-large has become the exact opposite of this ethos. Highly processed foods, genetically modified produce, and meat pumped with hormones are the most accessible food sources, and toxic chemicals like Roundup are used for maximum agricultural production. The companies that mass-produce your produce only care about monetary profit, increasing value for their shareholders, and extracting as much production from the planet as possible—your health is their disadvantage, not their priority. Most corporations make their food packaging flashy, affordable, and accessible; and in turn the chemicals in their foods make us sick, mentally wrecked, and unable to focus. For example, the company that made Roundup is Monsanto. In 2018, Monsanto was bought by Bayer, one of the world's largest pharmaceutical companies. This means that the same company that mass produces toxic chemicals for increasing food production is the same company that creates pharmaceutical medications, like SSRIs, benzodiazepines, and chemotherapy treatments. If you eat their food, you're most prone to take their "medicines." These medications temporarily resolve symptoms of mental dysregulation, but ultimately even further destabilize people out of their natural state of being due to the catastrophic impacts of the low-quality and excessive quantity of what they produce.

While using pharmaceutical medications can be and is essential for many, I encourage you to give yourself the gift of connecting with Indigenous-inspired wisdom teachings and nature-based practices that will create long-term health. That's not to say you need to or should want to stop Western forms of medicine and healing—that's a decision that only you can make. But living in full devotion to connecting with your own roots, and the root issues buried deep below the surface, you'll begin to find resolution for the things that cause you mental distress.

### *The Three Sisters*

A garden may be tended to by a single person, but it takes a community for it to thrive. It needs bees, ants, and hummingbirds for pollination. It needs the right natural fertilizer, in the right amounts, at the right times so the garden has fresh fuel to grow. When the winds come and the rain falls, the fertile soil can soak up the water and the roots will withstand the storms. There are underground networks of mushrooms that provide essential nutrients and carve out pathways so the roots have new places to deepen and take hold. The sun provides the energy for photosynthesis, like a fire that transforms a garden from little sprouts to abundant, life-giving stalks. Anything worth anything is done as a collaboration, and just like a garden, your mental health is no different.

The Native peoples of the Americas were intrinsically connected to the planet and each other, and lived in much greater wholeness than we do in our contemporary society. They knew how to forage for herbal remedies and also create thriving gardens, when to plant, and what plants to grow together. The Ancient people of Mesoamerica were the first to domesticate squash, maize (corn), and beans. In time, they learned how perfectly these plants worked together and called these the Three Sisters. A geographer called this trio "a symbiotic plant complex without an equal elsewhere." These ancient peoples created small mounds of dirt and planted maize on top of the mound. The maize provided a trellis for the beans to grow, and squashes were planted between the many mounds. Beans hold nitrogen in their root nodules, which stabilize the maize in high winds. The wide leaves of the squash plant shaded the ground, keeping the soil moist and helping prevent the growing of non-beneficial weeds. As you can see, this is a simple but incredible intelligence, one that yielded an abundance of high-quality crops, far more than could be grown via modern methods of crop rotation and mono-crop farming. Just like the Three Sisters, there are holistic ways of being and methods of healing that will assist you in creating an interconnected, abundant life full of gratitude.

By reading this book and devoting yourself to the practices within, seeking mental health support, having an organic-based diet, tending to your inner gardens daily, and surrounding yourself with an uplifting community, you will develop the mental fortitude to withstand the harmful stories or actions of others, any negative self-criticism, and feeling like your mind isn't a safe place. In your mind-garden, you can cultivate life-nourishing, loving thoughts, and like compost, turn any overwhelm from fearful thinking into fuel for a luscious life. Becoming aware of and lovingly tending to your thoughts, feelings, and emotions is good medicine for how you're growing and what you wish to cultivate. Only when you feel safe to feel things fully, and truly feel that being in your body is a good place to be, can you be healthy in your mind. By harnessing the power of your attention and intention, you will become the empowered creator of your reality.

### *You're Never Alone*

A healthy and vibrant imagination is respected and revered by the Maya. Medicine women and men, traditionally known as Aj Q'ij, or "spiritual guide," and also known as shamans, gain their powers from visionary spaces and their imagination, and learn from the unseen realms how to heal themselves, others, and their community. By developing your imagination, you open up to magical possibilities and can create the life of your dreams. As a child, I used my imagination to cope with difficult feelings, thoughts, and emotions, and it served me well. I have many pleasant memories because of the vivid imagery I created in my mind. This provided me an escape from the unstable and unsafe environment I was born into that is common for households of first- and second-generation immigrants. Harnessing my imagination was a gift. However, as I matured, it was important for me to recognize that it could be used as a coping mechanism if I was still unable to be fully present.

My suffering was compounded by the fact I was often neglected and ignored, something I know I am not alone in experiencing. Also, I often saw my caretakers, like my grandparents, mother, and stepfather, violently argue, and I saw other things that no child should see. My go-to imagined, alternate reality was that one day a loving and caring aunt from afar would scoop me up, adopt and save me, and we would live happily ever after. I could take dance lessons, not be poor, and not see my caretakers fight, be inebriated, or under the influence of harmful drugs. Another fantasy I played out is that my biological father, who left when I was just a baby, would come back and make everything right. These alternate realities rooted themselves in the fertile soil of my developing consciousness. It took me many years, lots of coaching, mentorship, and therapy, and a conscious reconnection with my true self—beyond the childhood pain—to fully accept my present reality. Only then did I find peace of mind.

However, I struggled with my mental health and other health issues throughout my teens and 20s because I didn't know how to self-soothe, regulate my nervous system, or seek help. I suffered in silence for most of my life. Sometimes I vented to friends or just completely numbed out. In a society that prizes a do-it-yourself mentality, being connected to a health-based community wasn't a priority, nor was seeking help. It simply wasn't a viable option for me back then because I had no reference for it. While it can seem hard to "do the work" to cultivate healing, the suffering of ignorance is truly much worse. Once you set out on a path of awakening and healing, you can't look back. You can't unsee the truth, but you can always go as slow as you need to and be as gentle as possible as you walk back home to yourself.

Looking to Indigenous ways, we see that it is natural for others to support our health in the seen and unseen worlds. To have a sense of community that supports our growth is not only healthy, but it's essential. Intimate connection to all aspects of Mother Nature via plants, animals, and all of life keeps us in balance and in harmony. Just like the Three Sisters growing, supporting, and thriving together, we are meant to do things with others—to live together, to raise our young together, to celebrate together, to grieve together, and to heal together. Nothing in nature grows in isolation. Only in laboratories are things grown on their own. However, it's solely up to you to put in the work to find healing, be it through therapy, coaching, mentorship, or nature-based practices. I recommend trying all of those and seeing what feels most supportive. Personally, I alternate the kinds of support I receive, but having a mentor is always a good idea. If you are like me, and do not have a relative or elder that you were particularly connected to that you could speak freely with and gain support from, I highly recommend seeking a mentor.

### *"Good Vibes Only" Doesn't Work Anymore*

Your mind can be a tricky thing. It's part of your body, yet sometimes it may feel like it's its own entity that does the thinking for you. However, you are not your mind. You are not your thoughts. Your thoughts do not define you, but they are your responsibility to become aware of. You also have the power to change the content, tempo, and tone of your thoughts, to notice when a negative thought pops up, think more positively, and give yourself an alternative way of thinking when needed. Unless we reprogram our thoughts to think more positively, our mind-chatter can be incessant and fueled with negativity from beliefs that were formed during our younger years when our minds were more malleable.

Our minds have been programmed to look for trouble and negativity, and so it is our responsibility to change the program. This is less about doing and more about witnessing. When we reprogram ourselves with compassion, we can develop trust and safety within ourselves. The word *compassion* means "to be with suffering." Therefore, instead of looking to "do" something about the thoughts we are having, the pain we feel, or the suffering we are experiencing, the key is to simply be with it. This presence with our pain allows us to take back our power and work with our mind and body instead of feeling like they are working against us. When we give away our power and allow the mind to run the show, it defaults on threat detection and fear-based thinking. Once we retake our place as witness of the mind, we will see with the eyes of the heart. This means we can see with clear vision and loving perspective, not only what the mind thinks, but in coherence with our body, heart, and soul.

Your mind wants to protect you. It says, "Watch out," or "Don't trust this." That may have seemed helpful up until a point, but now you get to take your power back by choosing to move out of fear and into trust. It may seem cliché, but you must choose to remember that throughout an ordinary day, you are safe, you can trust, and fundamentally, all is well even when things have seemed, or still seem, deeply unsettling. To change your life, you have to change your thoughts. This does not mean ignoring or bypassing challenging experiences and your emotions that come from them. Changing your thoughts is a complex process, but there are some subtle yet monumental shifts that can simplify it for you.

Most psychiatric methods, coaching modalities, and self-help books are based on moving you from a negative state into a more positive state. This creates a conflicting polarity, which is actually the fundamental root of all suffering. For example, if you feel fear, the opposite is feeling confident. Therefore, if you focus only on becoming confident but never identify the reason why you're feeling fear in the first place, the root cause of the fear will continue to manifest in your life. It's my desire that by reading this book, integrating the wisdom within, and applying these practices to your life, you will begin to identify what is on the other side of conflicting desires like fear and love, stress and peace, or scarcity and abundance. I'll give you a hint. What's on the other side is not another thing, but rather a state of being. And the greatest state of being? Gratitude.

What's truly transformative is not only cultivating the ability to identify an opposite positive thought, memory, or experience, but to revisit the original negative thought or memory to find what essential information it can offer you now. When thoughts that you do not want to think arise and bring feelings of self-doubt, judgment, shame, guilt, and the like, instead of ignoring it or smothering it with a positive thought, pause to question why you're thinking it, and you'll be shown something that needs your acknowledgment.

It's critical to not only have a preference for positive thoughts and avoid negative thoughts, but to choose to see that difficult experiences are often some of the greatest chances to evolve and become empowered. By giving yourself the time and space to connect with yourself, you will become "big" enough to witness both negative and positive things. By acknowledging negative thoughts without being influenced by them or preferring positive thoughts, you can take back your power by making intentional choices and not remain a victim to life's happenings.

The best time to practice this is when you fall asleep and immediately when you wake up. My waking practice includes feeling gratitude before I get up for my day. But sometimes, if I've had some really intense or sad dreams, I feel funky and I can't shake the feeling. I know that this is not permanent, yet when I wake up grumpy, my thoughts may become negative. So, I can begin my day with negativity and spiral in that downward direction, or I can tune in and understand that I'm thinking in a way that doesn't feel good to me. I've learned to stay with the feeling of grumpiness and compassionately be with it without needing to change it. First, I observe the negative thoughts I'm thinking. Then, I ask myself what it is that I wish to feel; this is identifying the opposite positive thought. Next, I notice how I feel thinking both of those thoughts at the same time. Once I am in tune with both kinds of thoughts, I will take action to acknowledge, express, or release what I'm thinking or feeling.

The most essential part is to prioritize gratitude. Identifying things I am grateful for, I will list at least three things like, "I am grateful for my home," "I am grateful to wake up this morning alive," or "I am grateful for my legs that can take me wherever I'd like to go." Then, I often find it helpful to move my body, so I'll play music that feels good, dance, or exercise. After observing my thoughts, feelings, and overall state, through physical movement, my state changes everything and I feel like myself again. If I just go straight to movement and begin my day without giving myself time to process my negative or positive thoughts, anxiety will linger around no matter what I do to bury it.

It is important not to shame yourself for feeling negatively or thinking negative thoughts. We are dualistic, dynamic human beings; we are not always angels. We are humans meant to experience ups and downs. We are ever-changing and multifaceted, so when you have moments that you would rather not experience, give yourself the time to become present and be without judgment. Use that as an opportunity to reflect and be with yourself, knowing that this too shall pass.

### *Self-Regulating*

When something is said that feels hurtful, regardless of if it was said on purpose or not, and we are not in a mental place to be curious, we tend to create a story in our mind. We can either become curious and ask questions or make our own determinations. For example, I've believed that people have been intentionally mean, that they are unsafe, and they've become my enemy. In the not-so-distant past, I have often gone into what I call "that is it" mode, where I am reactionary, and nothing else feels true except for my own mental story and subjective perspective. In the most intense of times, I was ready to run from the situation or relationship so the pain would end. In "that is it" mode, I have said things that are hurtful and harsh to defend and protect myself. When the story that I am unsafe, feel rejected, and am unloved has taken over my mind, I can't focus on what truly matters to me. Instead, I feel overwhelmed, my nervous system is dysregulated, and I am out of alignment with my truth. In this state I am not curious, trusting, or present.

The antidote is creating safety for myself, recognizing that I need a moment to regulate my nervous system so I can come back into my body. While alone, I give myself the time and space to shift my mind and body into coherence so that my thoughts don't run off with a story that isn't the whole truth. Then, I begin to feel safe in my body by listening to what I really need. Focusing on my breath, I relax and regulate my nervous system. I may use essential oils, I may go outside and place my feet on the grass (refer to the Embodiment Practice in Chapter 7), or I may drink a warm cup of cacao.

If my thoughts were racing, I am now more able to let go of trying to understand them or believe them. Once my mind has become focused, I can soften into the memory that I am hurt about something and that my feelings get to be validated. Then, I let myself feel my feelings. That means allowing myself to feel comfortable to be in my body amid sadness, blame, anxiety, anger, loneliness, and/or grief. None of your emotions are bad or wrong; they are your teachers and are supportive in bringing you back into alignment.

Once I am present, I work with somatic or embodiment practices and process my emotions. I will shake my body to release any energy that may be pent up. If I am feeling anger, I will do a rage ritual, and then move into a dance to feel present in my body and completely transmute any residual feelings (refer to the Embodiment Practice in Chapter 8). Also, simply going for a long walk always calms my mind. When we walk, our brains' left and right hemispheres come into balance.

Another simple yet powerful practice you can do right now to regulate yourself is to make the "voo" sound. This helps to stimulate the vagus nerve, which activates the parasympathetic nervous system, often called the "rest and digest" process. The "voo" sound can be practiced anytime you'd like to feel calmer. Simply inhale through your nose and on the exhale, make a deep and guttural "voo" for at least three counts. Extend your exhale of "voo" for as long as feels comfortable. Allow the sound to vibrate through your belly and whole body. Imagine the vibration giving you an internal relaxing massage that not only grounds and relaxes you, but also resets you. Doing this practice for about three minutes helps to soften our attachment to needing to logically understand or rationalize a painful feeling or event. This is also a helpful practice after experiencing or revisiting traumas or triggers.

Trauma isn't only about what did happen but also what didn't happen during our experience, limiting us from self-regulating or shifting into a harmonious state. The roots of our triggers and unwanted feelings and behaviors stem from our childhood trauma and/or generational trauma—the transmission of trauma from one generation to another, often as a result of significant traumatic events that impact an entire group or community. Therefore, as you cultivate mental health, it's essential to recognize that all your triggers are legitimate because they are tied to unresolved past traumas. Whether they seem big or small, they can all have an impact depending on how they show up in your memories and in your body. Whenever you feel scared, unstable, or insecure, you're unconsciously reverting to identifying with a younger version of yourself. Yet when you take ownership of your experience in the present moment, you can recognize that triggers are simply information your body hasn't yet been able to integrate. They give you an opportunity to move through something that has and still causes you pain.

Your daily triggers, big or small, are breadcrumbs in your journey of awakening. While they might seem bothersome or insignificant, addressing and healing these traumas can pave the way for a profound and gratitude-filled life. Your present behaviors mirror your development in earlier years, so by recognizing your actions, you can shift unhelpful patterns, evolve, and liberate yourself from old versions of who you have been. These patterns will continue to show up until we learn how to respond differently and consciously break the pattern or cycles that we are done repeating.

To break a pattern, you can't approach it with the same level of consciousness that created it. By creating safety in the body and self-regulating your emotions as they arise in the ways I've just shared, you pave the way for mental peace, bodily harmony, and the evolution of your soul. You do this by slowing down when you are in a situation where you would have previously gone into a default mode of people pleasing, fought back, or ran from the situation. Instead, you'll now breathe, notice how your body feels, and become aware of the present moment. Feel how you are safe in your body, know that you are safe to express your truth, and take time for yourself before you respond.

Thankfully, we are not defined by our mind or our thoughts. When you harness the full power of your mind as outlined in this chapter, you can use your imagination to manifest a beautiful inner and outer world. Using your imagination intentionally, combined with the power of gratitude, is an alchemical process, transforming even the most painful and traumatic of experiences into essential lessons in your process of healing, awakening, and blissful living. Aligning your mental power with the creative forces of the Universe, you will create a magic-filled life. This is using real magic to bring gratitude into every aspect of your life.

When you reprogram yourself by holding space for both the information of negative thoughts, the power of positivity, and then take intentional actions to feel gratitude, you become fully alive, fearing nothing, and live fully empowered. It takes practice to live life gratefully. It takes recognizing that the good, bad, positive, negative, painful, and uncomfortable are essential aspects to transform your way of being. Feeling deeply grateful regularly will nourish you from the inside out. The fruits you create will be vibrant and abundant, and your mind-garden will be a place of unconditional peace and the source of your prosperity.

### *Embodiment Practice: Speaking Mantras*

Words are incredibly powerful. We are casting spells with our words when we think, speak, or write them. Consider mantras. They are intentional phrases that you can repeat frequently in order to condition your mind to feel more trusting and safer on a regular basis.

Speak the following mantra three times: "All things are happening for my greatest good. Maltyox!" This can be said throughout the day, with your morning practice, whenever you're feeling overwhelmed, after dealing with difficult thoughts, or after the "voo" vagus nerve practice. You can also add more to your mantra like, "I am supported. I am safe. I am secure," or "I feel loved. I feel worthy. I feel blessed," or "In gratitude, I trust."

Use mantras on a daily basis for when you'd like to remember uplifting, empowering thoughts. Also, the word *maltyox* is an ancient and powerful word that I highly recommend adding to your mantras and daily life. Essentially, *maltyox* means "thank you" in the native K'iche' Mayan language, but this word carries much more meaning than just a simple thanks. When the Maya express this deeply felt thank you, they know it reaches from their hearts to the Heart of all things. Therefore, when you repeat this ancient word, do so fully with your heart and know that you are using a powerful vibration to infuse gratitude into your mind, body, and soul.

After saying the mantra, find a song that uplifts your mood (for inspiration, go to my Gratitude playlist @lifefullycolored on Spotify). By listening to music that makes you feel joyful, you will feel the medicine of the music, the magic of the mantra, and you will be glowing with gratitude.

Ask yourself, "What would life look like for all things to always be happening for my greatest good?" Imagine that. Embody that. What would it feel like? What would you see? Where would you be? Who would you be with?

Who will you become when you express this level of trust, safety, imagination, and gratitude every single day? Read the next chapter to find out, because your soul is calling you home.

CHAPTER 3:

# Soulful and Full of Soul

*"The soul has been given its own ears to hear things the mind does not understand."*

— Rumi

We come from something much bigger than what we see, something that connects us to the web of life, something mysterious and magical. We are humans, full of primal urges, feral tendencies, and animalistic behaviors. We are also beings—a divine essence that is immaterial, immortal, and ever present. It is this beingness, our soul, that through the vessel of the human body, weaves the web of our life together. Our soul comes from the Divine and is one with Great Spirit, weaving with and as the Great Weaver.

You are here on purpose, for a purpose. That purpose can extend as deep or surface as you choose. You can choose to believe that you don't have a purpose or that it's not something to search for. You can feel that sometimes you know your purpose and other times that you don't. It may be crystal clear and highly specific, or it can be fluid and ever-changing. Regardless of the depth of connection you have to your divine purpose or the beliefs you have, the truth is you are a soul having a human experience on this planet. Your soul is here to evolve and be the unique expression of divine love. While it's that simple, how your soul evolves is a highly complex, interwoven process that is influenced by your parents, childhood environments, the events surrounding your birth, your actual birthing process, and even the energetics during your conception as an egg and sperm. Then, as you age, there are millions, or if you're over the age of 33, billions of moments that influenced you in your process of learning more about yourself.

In the face of constant influence, by trusting your inner compass and authentically expressing your true self, you'll embody the unique soul essence that makes you, you. In this way, you will fulfill your purpose, understand the nuances of conditional love, and unlock the path to love unconditionally. Love the totality of who you are as a multidimensional being and become a living testament to divine expression of love that is you.

The more you interact with the worlds around you, you'll become increasingly diverse and distinct. Traveling the world to explore and honor other cultures, reconnecting with your ancestry, seeking out experiences that expand your awareness, and being curious about people outside of your sphere of comfort will age you like fine wine. Your ability to evolve, especially through difficult experiences, coupled with the courage to venture beyond your comfort zone and explore the unknown, will add depth and richness to your soul. We admire those who reach out into the Great Mystery, daring to explore the places most avoid, find the real soul of something, and do their part to further weave the Great Tapestry of Life. While every single human being has the potential, it is a choice to be soulful and full of soul—touching, even if only for passing moments, true liberation, real power, and discovering boundless gratitude for life. For it is gratitude that is the golden thread that will weave your body, mind, and soul, and thus your entire life, into wholeness.

### *Life School*

If you do not find your own sense of freedom from the world you're born into, the primal urge to survive within it will keep your soul at that level of evolution. This relates to you being born into a certain family, culture, and as a human on the planet. As an infant, your caregivers are how and what you learn about the world. Then, as you age, you begin to find more of yourself in the worlds around you. Your family dynamics are like the micro, while culture, religion, and the planet are the macro. Therefore, we take on the names we are given, the identities of culture we're born into, and place labels to try and understand the mystery of who and where we are. To do so is beautiful, critical even. However, if our identity is only as deep as the external aspects of ourself, our soul will become suffocated by the labels and masks, forgetting that before there was a named, structured world, all things came from the Great Mystery.

Being born into dysfunctional households usually results in having conflicting bonds with abusive, neglectful, narcissistic, or unconscious parents. This pattern of bonding with unhealthy dynamics will then play out in adulthood until our soul can't take it anymore. We must do the work to learn more about ourselves, how to evolve, and how to return to our soul's unique expression. As adults, we have the power of choice and the freedom to live without needing to please others for survival. However, many people get into work environments and romantic relationships that perpetuate unresolved codependent tendencies. If we let it, what we experience in childhood and adolescence is like a warm-up for when we have the power to choose for ourselves. Our parents are simply part of the assignment that our soul chose to learn in "Life School." Having compassion and forgiveness for our parents allows us to be liberated from bonds we've created with them.

We are no longer the vulnerable children we once were. We can stop looking to others to love or accept us once we realize that ultimately our soul is untarnished by the workings of this world. It is our body that keeps record of the pains we face and the pleasures we seek. Our soul is infinite, perfectly divine, and one with Spirit, yet it's here to have a human experience. We simply must do our best to be aligned with our unique expression and purpose of being a perfect expression of love in a seemingly imperfect world. It only takes a single moment of intention to connect with your soul and reclaim your birthright of bliss. By doing so, you remember your place in the web of life.

### *The Dance between Grief and Gratitude*

Well into my adult life, I learned that my father was far from who I believed him to be. I knew he had a tragic life, yet I imagined that he was a kind man, and that if only we could have been connected, everything would be better. I felt guilty that I never got to tell him I loved him one last time or even tell him good-bye. After he died by suicide when I was 22, I blamed myself and others for not putting me in connection with him sooner. I believed I forever missed my chance to connect with a father figure of my dreams. Because of this, I continued the fantasies I had as a child of being rescued, and in turn, wished I could have rescued him. This can be a thrilling but unhealthy way of seeing the world, one where we and others remain victims in our life's story. The truth is that he didn't want to be connected to me, and for a good reason. Roughly 12 years after his death, I learned that my father was abusive. His abandonment, which seemed like a tragedy for my entire life, turned out to be a blessing in disguise. For this, I am grateful.

However, grief and gratitude are interwoven together; fullness of gratitude comes from our ability to grieve deeply. The process of grieving is not linear, and it comes in waves. I grieve for those he hurt, deeper enmeshed in the pain he caused and more directly burdened by the weight of his actions. As someone who has been harmed as a child, a teen, and an adult, I know the pain and confusion that comes with being violated. While I am grateful to have not experienced abuse from my father, it has taken time to heal from abuse by others along with the wounds from his abandonment. Choosing to not remain a victim of what has happened to me, I've done the unthinkable by opening up to considering that all things happen for me. Sometimes we have no idea why things unfold the way they do, but ultimately all things are always happening for our greatest good, for our soul's evolution, and the fulfillment of our sacred purpose.

Everything is divinely orchestrated, and all experiences can support our soul's journey through life. I love that truth because it empowers me to take radical responsibility for what is mine to grieve, heal, transmute, and let go of. We also live in a mysterious world where harmful, devastating, and destructive events happen for no good or apparent reason. For years, I ran away from the ways

I'd been hurt and numbed myself from feeling pain fully. Fantasizing about a different, better life, reality eventually caught up with me. Once it did, I realized that when life breaks our heart open, we can put up walls and harden our heart, or alchemize our pain and let it fuel us in a higher purpose than we ever could have imagined trying to do it all on our own. Since we are the creators of our own reality, we can choose our truth for ourselves. What feels more empowering, actively choosing to see that life happens to you or for you? Which truth would you like to claim for yourself?

When we are connected to our soul, we emanate and are able to express love. We will not be able to do this at every given opportunity, and that's okay. But we have the sacred responsibility to course-correct when we go off path. It takes practice and actively remembering that the suffering of being unconscious is much worse than the struggle of doing the work to stay balanced and in alignment. The more we act from a place of pain and become disconnected, the more we veer away from love. When we are disconnected from our soul, we perpetuate separation, hate, and abuse, even in the most subtle of ways. Feeling separate is not your or anyone's natural state of being. It is learned in this lifetime or another, yet it's a part of your human story via familial, generational, cultural, or societal patterning.

For example, I learned that my father was five years old when a Catholic priest harmed him. From this trauma, he learned how to hurt others, and he grew further disconnected. After he and my mother conceived me, he began taking drugs, which put him into further fragmentation. He was very smart, a prolific reader and writer, and had an ability to influence others. Because of this, he even started a prominent gang. He was in and out of prison, and as I previously mentioned, he eventually took his own life. When he did so, I was devastated.

When we are disconnected and fragmented, we are suffocating our soul's expression. We may be learning valuable lessons by staying in dark places, but we're unable to sustainably feel joy, gratitude, and spread love. Instead, we are vibrating at a low frequency that keeps us stuck. Numbing ourselves to avoid the pain of being disconnected to our truth and the Divine will leave us with a nagging feeling. Many people will live their entire lives with this unresolved sense of disconnect that may only be felt as loneliness, despair, or depression.

While it can seem difficult—even impossible at times—it's essential that we shine light on even the most difficult of our experiences. Why? Only then can we alchemize them and use them to *fuel* us in our purpose. It is possible to return to our soul's purpose no matter how fragmented we have become, yet we must choose this for ourselves. That is in our scope of possibility, and while it's an incredibly empowering choice, it's entirely up to us. Otherwise, we'll miss the opportunity to transform. You know you're alive right here, right now, so make the absolute most of it.

### *The Most Beautiful Truth of All*

At the end of my 20s, I was in the deepest pain of my life. I was disconnected from my soul, but my heart knew there was more to life than what I saw around and felt within me. I had glimpsed true beauty and magic before, usually in nature, but it always seemed fleeting. I loved animated movies, vintage things, puppies, fairies, mystical realms, and romance, and while these externally provided a sense of pleasure, it was never enough to change my life.

I also had a lifelong vivid imagination that allowed me to tap into magic within me, but again, it never lasted long enough to fix anything.

Unfortunately, I was in a downward spiral—in what is often called the "dark night of the soul." I spent a few years seemingly stuck in the same life doing the same things. Yet, buried underneath it all, I knew something else existed. I retained a glimmer of hope and revived my ability to imagine. That was all I needed to get started.

I imagined what could be and started taking steps to live a better life, manifesting a new reality. It started with simply following my bliss and what felt good for my soul. However, moving out of the dark night of the soul was not the end of my pain. I still repeated unhealthy patterns and continually moved through different layers of healing. The process of coming home to our true self is a positive spiral, and healing is never reaching a destination but a dynamic journey. This spiral can either have a downward trajectory, burying our soul under diseases and disorders, or it can be positively charged, ever expanding and growing our ability to give and receive love, regardless of circumstances.

Depending upon what we learn in this wild and wondrous world, we can either get further from or closer to our soul's unique truth. Sometimes getting to the lowest low can help shake us out of our suffering so we can take the steps to reconnect with our soul. Like being woken from a bad dream, it isn't fun to be shaken awake, but it breaks the spell of what isn't real anymore.

In 2018, I was a yoga teacher, yet I still didn't know who I truly was. I was in Phase One, or what I like to call the "Love and Light" phase—also known as spiritual bypassing. This is where everything is rainbows and butterflies, and we gloss over our pain because we do not have the capacity or the tools to feel safe enough to sit with deep and heavy emotions. Once we learn how to self-regulate and finally give ourselves the time and space to feel things fully, unafraid to make or become an emotional mess, we naturally move out of this heavy process. There is healing found after a really good cry, a really hard laugh, or a deep cathartic release. There's a special sweetness in the sigh you make after giving yourself the gift of doing something difficult but good for your soul.

After feeling badly for years about something, be it loneliness, fear, or unhappiness, and likely making ourselves feel bad for feeling bad, and then finally experiencing what it's like to feel good, we often crave and depend on feeling good. This creates the conflicting polarity that I spoke of in Chapter 2. When we feel unhappy, the logical thing to want is to feel happy. When we feel lonely, the logical thing is to want to feel loved. Alas, the great work of your life is to be able to recognize when you're caught in these conflicting desires. Exploring the roots of the negative part, surrendering attachment to only experiencing the positive parts. Opening your heart, which is easy to say and hard to do, will lead you into a state of being aligned with your soul's true essence. The more you practice this, the less you'll get stuck or be swept away by your feelings. Your soul gently asks, and sometimes intensely demands, that you develop the emotional safety to fully feel your painful emotions. This is how you become the cycle breaker and the healer of your life and lineage.

You will make mistakes, get some bumps and bruises, and become forgetful again. You may even enter another dark night of the soul. Yet the next time you enter into the depths of darkness, you'll do so with more confidence because you'll have the tools to remember what's true. You will remember that the fullness of gratitude comes after feeling grief fully, and your soul will remember your connection to all things. You will remember that you are never alone—your Ancestors, Mother Nature, and Great Spirit will always be there to guide you. Be easy on yourself when you forget, slip up, or make mistakes. Yes, you are a perfect soul, but in this human form, you are perfectly imperfect. And to me, that is the most beautiful truth of all.

### *CholQ'ij: The Sacred Mayan Calendar*

Ancient Mayan mathematicians and astrologers decoded reality by identifying the patterns, cycles, and predominant energies that influence us as human beings. Since most of the ancient codices and records were systematically destroyed by conquistadors, colonizers, and Catholic priests, much of the Mayan wisdom teachings that remain are incredibly simplistic, highly abstract, or difficult to comprehend. But after connecting with my roots and Mayan lineage, it's become my life's work to bridge Mayan wisdom from the Mesoamerican jungles to the concrete jungle.

One part of Mayan cosmovision and cosmology that is easier to understand is the sacred Mayan Calendar. Also known as the CholQ'ij, this tool can support you in discovering your soul's purpose, the arc of your evolution, and accurately define your unique personality. The calendar is based upon the same mathematics that created the Universe, and the fact it still remains is a blessing. Your Mayan birth chart, which comes directly from the CholQ'ij and is called a Tree of Life reading, will support you in discovering your soul's purpose.

When someone claims to have found their purpose, they're likely speaking to the fact that they have discovered their dharma. Dharma is an important Vedic concept that refers to your duty and sacred mission in life, and while Mayan elders speak at length about this concept, a succinct word for it has not yet been found. Another word for this is *ikigai*, which comes from Okinawa, Japan, and means "something that gives a person a sense of purpose and a reason for living." Understanding dharma, along with karma and your persona, will liberate your soul and connect you to your true self. However, to discover your dharma, you must first be aware of your karma and your persona.

Karma is another Vedic theory relating to the reincarnation of your soul. Karma speaks to the effect of your individual actions, extending from past lives to your present and future lives. This theory speaks to the universal principle that all actions you make have a beneficial or non-beneficial result. The word *karma* literally means "action," and when you actively work on yourself to become aware of your behaviors, you will see positive changes. This is the cause-and-effect principle in action.

It's important to note that karma is a theory, and the only way to prove if it's true is by taking intentional action to positively influence your reality. It's your awakening that becomes the proof if you're cultivating "good" karma or clearing "bad" karma. If karma is real, and the theory of cause-and-effect holds up; every bit of your joy or suffering is part of your karmic responsibility because it is showing up in your reality. Your current reality is a reflection of your past, and how you now respond is a reflection of your future. Therefore, you must make decisions to positively influence your reality and those around you, and in doing so, you'll activate your soul's divine purpose.

One of the many things I have learned by my teacher, Nana Lu, is that the Maya believe each soul becomes a human with a unique karma and that it comes to this planet so it can evolve. They theorize that if you die past 80 years old, you will become one with the Cosmos. By working through your karma and having strong personal integrity, you may become a tree, an element like the wind, a butterfly, or even a star, working with and as the forces of the Cosmos without any sense of separation. If and when you work through your karma, it's believed you will not come back as a human on this planet. Those who choose to not awaken or don't evolve in accordance with their soul's purpose will be reincarnated. The Maya also believe if someone does dishonorable things, they will come back as something less favorable than being a human, like a rat or an unhoused dog. If someone dies in an accident, they will come back with similar situations so that they can transcend that experience. While much of this is impossible to prove, there is no harm caused in doing all you can to make your world and the lives of those around you better.

Your persona, or personality, also significantly influences your soul's evolution. Personality comes from behavioral, cognitive, and emotional patterns given to you via biological and environmental factors such as your parents, ancestry, culture, and society. You're born with these interrelated patterns, and they're relatively stable, but they will shift throughout your lifetime. Ultimately, you take on a personality to cope and merge with the environments you're born into. There are endless frameworks to understand your personality from astrology, Gene Keys, Myers-Briggs, Enneagram, and of course, the Mayan Tree of Life reading. While these are helpful and can significantly support your process of awakening, fundamentally, your persona is not you. Personality is the "you" that's influenced and motivated by the external environments you're surrounded by at birth, throughout adolescence, and as an adult, the person you portray to the world. Most humans are firmly identified with their persona as their true self, and while there is nothing wrong with this, it generates and perpetuates a lot of suffering. Learning to work through your karma and work with your persona are essential to live your soul's birthright of bliss.

I learned how to read the Mayan Calendar from one of my teachers, Tata Mark, and I learned that your Mayan Tree of Life reading is based on your birth date and time. This moment in time holds the keys to comprehensively understanding your karma and persona, and it unlocks your dharma! You have a predominant energy, your main Nawal, that stays with you your entire life. Your Nawal is your character and defines your life path. There are 20 Mayan Nawals, and in a reading, each Nawal combines with a number, 1 through 13. A Nawal and number together create a "Sign."

This reading also identifies your feminine and masculine aspects, as well as your past, present, and future. In total, you have nine Signs in your Tree of Life. You also have a Trecena, which is your emotional drive, and your Year Lord, which influences you on an instinctual level. If the number of your Year Lord is higher than your main Nawal, this energy will have a greater influence on you. Learning how all nine of your Mayan Signs in a Tree of Life reading, as well as your Trecena and Year Lord, all work together to help you learn who you are, why you are the ways that you are, where you've been, where you're headed, your weaknesses, and your strengths. Essentially, it outlines your dharma, karma, and persona.

The Mayan Calendar, and a Tree of Life reading, is based on sacred mathematics. Just think that thousands of years ago, they had the technology and awareness to know as much, if not more, about astronomy and astrology than we do today. If you look deeply into the Mayan cosmology, their calculations are based upon the same numbers used by the Vedic people, who accurately dated the age of the planet to around 4.32 billion years old; modern scientists claim that it's 4.5 billion years old. What's magical to consider is that the same math that accurately dated the age of the planet has been directly translated into the 20 Mayan Nawals, which hold the essence of all creation along with the 13 coordinating numbers. Since each person has a past, present, and future, as well as feminine and masculine aspects, and a predominant persona, when each of these parts are given a Sign based upon math that created the Universe itself, you're given a comprehensive look into the inner framework of your unique soul.

### *Soul Mission*

Your soul has a divine mission, and through karmic challenges you gain more awareness, opening up to your true self and your purpose. You can either work through this karma and evolve—or not. The persona you take on from what you experience in your malleable years can either be a key that unlocks your true self, or the thing that takes over and runs the show. It's your dharma that calls out to your heart to keep showing up and allows you to live out your divine mission. If you're disconnected from your soul, unaligned with your divine mission, and not working through your karma, you will feel a sense of loneliness. No matter how busy and distracted you keep yourself, you will feel something is amiss. If it's difficult to be alone with yourself, you're bound to feel lonely. There is nothing wrong with this, but it's simply a signal that you aren't in connection with your soul.

If you do not work toward constantly reconnecting with your soul, you will get further from living your purpose. Finding yourself in experiences that are testing you is one way to learn and evolve, but finding your truest self through bliss and ease is just as legitimate, healing, and valuable. Only you can devote yourself to reconnecting to your soul's essence. External situations, environments, relationships, and guidance are essential to support you living your purpose. However, if they are used as an escape or a crutch, no matter how much effort you put into living your dharma, a nagging emptiness will define your day-to-day life. You must integrate your persona and allow karma to work as your ally for your soul to live out its sacred purpose.

When you are connected to your soul, which only ever happens in the present moment, you can find gratitude for all experiences needed for your evolution. This opens you up to unconditionally loving yourself and others. This pure love and gratitude that is your soul's truest expression will extend into the world around you. If someone asks, "What can I do to save the world?" the truest answer is always, "Remain lovingly connected to yourself." A better question to ask is, "What must I do to live whole and complete within myself without any regrets?" Love yourself first so that the love you offer the world is sustainable. You cannot love wholly if you are not accepting or loving of all parts of your body, mind, and soul. When you feel connected, integrated, and soul-satisfied, with gratitude as a result, you will attract the right environments, opportunities, and relationships that aid you in the fulfillment of your purpose.

### *Embodiment Practice: Cosmic Light Meditation*

This is a practice you can do with yourself to feel aligned within your body, mind, and soul. I recommend recording yourself slowly reading the following paragraphs to guide yourself through this meditation or having someone read it to you. If you feel uncomfortable recording and listening to yourself, just remember, as long as you're alive, there's only one person you'll always be around: yourself. So, you might as well learn to love that person. You are a home for the eternal and undying spark of the Divine, and you get to learn to honor all parts of yourself as such . . . even if that means listening to yourself speak. Experiencing this practice, not just reading through it, will help remind you of who you truly are and what you're really here to do.

Come to a comfortable seat. Sitting cross-legged, roll your shoulders up, back, and down so that you are sitting up nice and tall, with a straight yet comfortable spine. Try to keep your back gently open and broad so energy flows freely through the back of your heart. Close your eyes. Take a few deep, relaxed breaths. Feel your belly soften, face soften, jaw and mouth soften, and allow your entire body to relax into this moment. Feel your body grounded into your seat, whether on the floor, cushion, or chair.

Next, begin to breathe into your heart, the seat of your soul. Use your imagination or feel, see, or sense a light that comes from your heart. Notice the light swirl or vibrate or glow around your heart. Now feel the light move down through your body until it reaches the base of your spine. From here, feel the light move down into the soils beneath you, into the rock and sediment, until it reaches the core of the planet, where a healing and unconditionally loving energy resides. On your next inhale, draw the energy up through your body, engulfing your whole being with this light. Feel the light move through you and out the top of your head. Feel or see the light shoot up into the Cosmos, and then circle back down into you. Remain here for some time.

Feel yourself being this middle point, this vessel, and the anchor of healing light energy between the planet and the Cosmos. Feel your body, mind, and soul wrapped within this cocoon of planetary and cosmic light. In time, as feels right for you, send out this light in every direction, bathing the entire planet with this light. Take notice of how you feel right here, right now. May you always remember, right when you need to, that you are the light.

Come back into your bodily awareness. Take a deep inhale and exhale audibly with any noise that you feel. Feel yourself fully grounded into your seat or cushion. Now, for the most important part, put your arms around yourself, wrapping yourself in your own loving embrace. Hug yourself for at least 30 seconds, giving and receiving your own love. Feel how safe you are with your own affection. Notice how much you can trust this love. You can soften into this loving embrace, relaxing the shoulders, and breathing into your heart. To end the practice, only when you feel ready and if you desire, go embrace someone or something you love! Could even be a tree or a houseplant. Take notice of how you feel after embrace something or someone else, and remember, you can always return home to embracing yourself. Because now, your soul knows your body and mind really are good places to be.

CHAPTER 4:

# It's Okay to Let Your Walls Down

*"People think a soul mate is your perfect fit, and that's what everyone wants. But a true soul mate is a mirror, the person who shows you everything that's holding you back, the person who brings you to your own attention so you can change your life."*

— Elizabeth Gilbert

Prioritizing a connection with body, mind, and soul is your essential foundation to relate to others from a place of love instead of fear. Since we experience trauma relationally, the most powerful way to learn about yourself and find deep healing is through relationships. However, relationships can be confronting. They can feel scary or edgy at times, but the triggers you allow yourself to feel and heal are what help you grow. An intimate relationship with a significant other can be the catalyst for some of our deepest healing, and healthy relationships with a therapist, confidant, community, support group, and/or spiritual guide will help you overcome walls you've built around your heart.

Having clear and strong boundaries is critical for all relationships, but boundaries set from a place of fear can keep us imprisoned and stagnant in our growth. We all make mistakes in relationships or have gotten into ones that aren't good for us; it can be a painful learning curve. But letting down your walls and simultaneously setting clear limits of what you will and will not allow creates relationships that support your growth. This chapter is essential, as it offers you a standard for how to interact with others around you. You'll learn the principles of reciprocity, how to set healthy boundaries and stick to them, and how to be the model of relationships you wish to see in the world.

Healing is meant to be done with others. We are meant to be supported by our kin, the planet, plants, animals, the Cosmos, and each other. We are meant to gather and grow together, sharing our gifts with each other. We are meant to live and thrive together. Feeling lonely or separated from any aspect of life creates sickness, as is seen in our current society with so many diseases of heart and mind. For too long, humanity has believed the lie that we are fundamentally separate from each other. All things are interconnected, whether we always see it or not. Our individual actions affect the whole, and we can work together to complement each other.

For thousands of years, humans have gathered for good times and for bad times. It is in our DNA to feel deep grief and celebrate boundless gratitude with each other. Connecting with those who really see and respect us allows us to feel healthy, happy, and whole. As a human species, we have lost our way of loving one another as sisters and brothers. We forget that first and foremost, we are one family, native to this planet. We forget that the deepest truth is that there are no strangers. So many people feel disconnected, and that has led them to lose their way and perpetuate violence, hate, or abuse in their search to be loved. Thus, every action you can make is either to love or to be loved. If you are deeply connected to the worlds within and around you, your focus will be on loving all things, and you will feel less inclined to do things in search of being loved.

In a state of giving love, you will not need others or things to fill a void. Objects, or objectifying others, will only keep you in a state of perceived separation and a cycle of suffering. You will not be able to take anyone or anything with you when your soul leaves your body. However, as you transcend this world, those who were connected to you will notice your absence. They will remember how you made them feel. Yet your ability to impact others stretches far beyond those who you know, sending ripples of energy with every person you're around. When you love a perceived stranger, it is to love an extension of your human family and live in right relation. This does not mean it's wise to blindly trust someone you know nothing about, because trust is earned. Yet, it does mean that when you're aligned with your natural instinct of loving first, you'll create the necessary boundaries and seek out opportunities to live in a way that honors your life and sovereignty.

### *The Mess Is the Magic*

Syris, my husband and co-author of this book, and I were joined together by Tata Izaias during Wayeb, one of the most sacred times for the Maya. Our union happened during a Mayan fire ceremony with Guatemalan volcanoes and the splendor of Lake Atitlán as our backdrop. It was pure magic. I adore Syris and treasure being his partner. But our relationship is not perfect. We brush up against each other's edges, and we show each other more to life than we could have found on our own. We hold the mirror of reflection up to one another, and every day, we must choose to love everything we see in ourselves and each other. What we show each other may irritate our shadows or trigger an untended wound, yet we choose to actively love one another. As a result, we can get through anything. At times, it feels like we are ideally matched since we have the same values, we enjoy the same activities, we eat similarly, and we prioritize our mental, physical, and spiritual health. Other times, it's obvious that we upset each other in ways only the other can. Both are medicine, and by choosing to have faith amid it all, we overcome fears and can find gratitude for all things.

Relationships aren't always easy. They can be messy and full of mistakes, yet they assist us in finding true love and ultimately, transcendence. A sense of safety, freedom, trust, and respect is essential. Without these, any relationship will not be sustainable, let alone support you in finding deeper layers of bliss, fulfillment, and love. Relationships are not just about the other person but about how you can explore and experience yourself as an embodiment of love. Being in a safe and empowering union is one of life's greatest gifts. It's also where the deepest self-work can happen, and like my Mayan elders, I also believe we are much more powerful when we have a loving partner during our life's journey. Syris and I have worked through so much within our union, and the first few years of our relationship were some of the most challenging of our lives. It hasn't always been a smooth or stable ride, but we've done our best, and our love continues to blossom.

Many of us haven't had truly healthy relationships modeled to us. We've had our fill of rom-coms and idealistic social media couples or families, which I have nothing against. But predominantly, Western culture has continually placed the feminine in the position of being swept off her feet rather than supported in growing her roots deeper, treated with unwavering compassion, or supported in both her majesty and her mess. Western religious systems have produced societies that lead to the feminine being steamrolled, their voices suppressed, and not being legitimately honored. Because of the abuse that the feminine has taken for thousands of years, in our current society, there are many examples of hyper-masculine women. There is absolutely nothing wrong with this. Each person should have the right to express themselves, their sexuality, and their energetic disposition however they feel. Yet as is true for all actions, when done from a place of compensation, fear, or hurt, it will only deepen a sense of separation.

What we all need is to feel whole and complete within ourselves, yet what many of us yearn for is to feel whole and complete through relationships. We must be gentle on ourselves and each other as we learn throughout the process of cultivating healthy relations. Trusting our hearts and choosing faith over fear will always lead us in the right direction.

### *Romance Is Not Always Roses and Rainbows*

Romantic relationships offer a profound opportunity to heal from past hurts and for our soul to evolve. Unhelpful behaviors will come creeping in at what seem like random times, yet these are opportunities for learning. It's healthy to have disagreements, moments of friction, and to butt heads. However, there are ways to constructively disagree and have conflict without blaming or villainizing the other. If you or your partner are emotionally dysregulated, it will inevitably lead to feelings of hurt, separation, and distress. It's so important that each of you take time to tend to your inner garden so you can seek resolution from a grounded place. For there to be healing, at least one partner must be regulated to hold the space for the other to express their feelings. This is why it is essential to create a partnership with someone you have similar values, beliefs, ideals, and goals with, so when you disagree, you can both prioritize respect, a desire to understand, and seek resolution instead of being "right."

Someone I once mentored mentioned how she and her now ex-husband never fought. On the outside, it seemed they had a transcendent and sacred union, and she felt they did as well. However, this is another example of the three phases I outlined in Chapter 1. For most of their marriage, they predominantly remained in Phase One, a phase defined by suppression. They created a level of peace and fulfillment that seemed to work for them but were simultaneously suppressing themselves and not valuing healthy conflict. They were both successful in their own businesses, which kept them busy and never fully vulnerable with each other even though she tried many times to explore deep, emotional places with her beloved.

Eventually, the suppression of Phase One erupted and was made obvious by her husband being wildly unfaithful due to his unresolved traumas, shame, and suppressed emotions. While it could be easy to think of him as the monster for cheating and her as the victim, ultimately, she could see how they both created an unhealthy dynamic. However, since there was no excuse for his actions of being unfaithful, she did the natural thing and moved the relationship fully into Phase Two by ending the relationship. This phase is defined by separation. Separation can feel like hell, and ultimately, it is if we stay there. When we feel separate, we're lonely, conflicted, and afraid. But in this phase, something magical happens. This is where we discover what we deserve, desire, and who it is we truly are. From separation, we either slip back into the suppression and unconscious behaviors of Phase One, or we emerge into the sweetness of Phase Three. In this transcendent place, we are free to be our true self and can welcome in true love.

Ideally, you want to find a partner who you can move into and through all three phases with. You deserve someone who will hold you in your fear, gently nudge you out of suppression, honor your heart's expression, and remind you of what's most true when you're feeling separate. Moving through the phases within yourself can be messy, and even more messy with another person. Conflict arises when someone feels their boundaries are being crossed or not being loved despite their mess.

It's important to remember that conflict is typical. Yet, you must pause and check in with yourself any time you are feeling dysregulated. It's essential to be with someone that you feel safe enough to not always be perfect for and can be in your overwhelm, mess, or intensity. However, and this is essential, if you begin to depend on others to get you out of these moments, it will also lead to major conflict within yourself and the relationship. This is why the practices from the previous chapters are offered first to help you self-soothe, self-regulate, and come into alignment. Even though Syris and I have had our fair share of suppression and separation, we've learned how to move to and through these phases, leading us into so much sweetness, within ourselves and each other.

### *Healthy Relationships 101*

In our romantic relationship, we want to be our true self. Personally, I have always prided myself on being authentically raw, wild, and real. In the beginning of our relationship, this way of being used to trigger Syris's way of being, which was perceptive, poised, and methodical. The things that attracted us to each other were also the things that could irritate us about each other the most. At times, I am loud, messy, and sassy in my feminine expression, and this would conflict with his masculine, structured, and oftentimes stubborn presence. By perceiving my sassy or loudness as being rude, he responded with a seriousness that triggered my wound of feeling like I was bad or wrong. Growing up, I was shamed for my feelings and how I expressed myself, and in the beginning of our relationship, I felt a similar sense of dread for just being myself.

Ultimately, Syris was able to expand his ability to hold space for me in my mess and my majesty, and I was called forward to observe my own wounds, shame, and unconscious behaviors. We worked through the fact that my behaviors, although a petty annoyance, were simply unconscious yet harmless behaviors since I was (usually) not directing my sassiness toward him. Furthermore, they were an opportunity for him to accept and love all of me and be called forward to support the feminine within himself, me, and others. In turn, I learned to be more gentle and graceful, while still retaining my authentic wild and raw self-expression. Instead of staying in Phase One by him suppressing his frustrations and me suppressing my expression, we moved into and through Phase Two by standing our ground, setting boundaries, and seeking resolution. This is the only way to reach the sweetness and true love that we all seek.

When we are children, the development of our nervous and endocrine (which regulates our hormones) systems are predominantly influenced by our parents and primary caregivers. As we age, the same pathways in our brain and body that we once used to feel safe and taken care of as children get repurposed as our attraction to romantic partners, certain friends, and those we look up to. It takes some time to fully see the things we dislike about others, but eventually, any unresolved traumas from our past are likely to be instigated through our relationships. We all have initial gut feelings if a relationship is good for us, but relationships are destined to become sweeter or to sour with time. In the beginning of romantic partnerships, in the "honeymoon phase," people statistically put in increased effort into their physical appeal, emotional availability, and mental flexibility. However, amid routines, shared belongings, and cohabitation, people may forget how sacred their relationship is.

Regardless of how established, promising, or incredible a relationship seems, it is a daily choice to stay in it. When people forget to honor themselves and lose themselves to the relationship, the relationship can take on an identity that is greater than the two people who came together to create it. Conversely, a relationship can be sidelined by it not being a priority due to partners focusing on living their own lives. The trick is to strike a healthy balance between sovereignty and self-sacrifice. Since relationships, like the humans that make them, are infinitely complex and ever-changing, you must handle situations with as much gentleness as possible, and request that others do the same. Only you can determine what you will or will not stick around for. But living in a culture that seems to offer hundreds or thousands of potential "connections" via dating apps, giving the illusion that there are endless options at your disposal, commitment to someone through challenges and conflict is true relational currency.

We cannot, nor should we try to change our partners. Seeing our partner's patterns is an opportunity to look into the mirror of our own ways and focus on what we want to change about ourselves. In many ways, Syris's mother was an angel in this life and still is for us after her passing. She was an extraordinary embodiment of gentleness and unconditional love toward her children, grandchildren and the children of many others, yet her married life was spent focusing on what she thought Syris's father needed to change. As their children, it was obvious to us that they both did things that crossed each other's boundaries and caused them deep distress. However, whenever they were advised to seek therapy or mental health support, neither one followed through, sticking to their own points of view that it was the other person who needed to change. She held this perspective up until her very last days, passing from leukemia much sooner than anyone that knew her expected. Leukemia is a cancer of the blood, a physical manifestation of prolonged dis-ease in her heart.

Moving through the grief of her passing and the celebration of her life allowed Syris and I to discover many ways we could learn from his Ancestors, choosing what we will or will not carry forward. In all of our relations, we have the sacred responsibility to heal from our generational and childhood patterning to co-create relationships that support us learning through grace, ease, love, and respect. By holding strong boundaries and simultaneously allowing our edges to be stretched, we can develop our compatibility, something many people never allow themselves to experience.

Another aspect of conflict that limits the development of compatibility is miscommunication and misunderstanding. The way that we interact and communicate with a partner can feel like we're speaking two different languages where one person doesn't know what the other means. We can work on translation and better communication, yet the saying, "Find someone who speaks your language, otherwise you will spend a lifetime trying to interpret your spirit," reminds us that even though we love someone dearly, we may not always be each other's person for the long run.

The beauty of being human is that we can learn from each other and integrate the lessons of moving through misunderstandings. The best way to do this is to become deeply curious and trust that even if you don't understand, by remaining open and asking questions, you're likely to feel more deeply what your partner is sharing. One of the best questions we can ask is, "What do you mean by that?" This question can be used in all kinds of relationships to find connection. When you're listening, I invite you to try and feel what they're saying rather than logically understand. Also, by reflecting back the word or phrase you sense is most important to someone after they've shared allows them to feel heard and understood. For example, if someone says, "My feelings are hurt by what you did," you can reflect, "I'm sorry your feelings are hurt and that my actions hurt you."

On many occasions, Syris and I have almost broken up, yet we made fundamental shifts and renewed ourselves, staying in the relationship. We have had such shifts, at times barely making it through, yet completely different on the other side. A part of us feels like we've died and are reborn, which is exactly what happens. We emerge with a deeper sense of honor and respect for the process of growth, for ourselves, and for each other.

Extraordinary, long-lasting, and healthy relationships are the products of intention, determination, and two people who are willing to continue leveling up together as one. Therefore, we must have things in common and enjoy each other's company, humor, intellect, and way of being. We want to adore the person that we are doing life with, so that when the challenges come, we will be able to find and follow the thread of gratitude that leads us back to love. Sometimes it feels as if there is a supernatural force that keeps us together. Some people call it God or destiny, but by devoting our lives to something much bigger than ourselves and to being open to its guidance, we make sacrifices when needed, hold our boundaries when that's needed, and have the humility to admit when we are wrong.

### *Practice Makes Imperfections Perfectly Okay*

Here is a practice Syris and I have used to overcome fears, miscommunications, and truly get to the heart of our union. First, once both partners feel grounded and openhearted, the partner that is seeking to be heard speaks. The other partner listens without interrupting unless it's to simply ask for a rephrase or further explanation. The speaking partner first offers their fears/feelings. It's critical to speak on fears and feelings using "I" statements and refrain from making their feelings about the other.

For example, "I feel hurt by what you did," is a more resonant way to speak rather than, "I feel you hurt me." Saying "you hurt me" places the emphasis on the action rather than the emotion, which might come across as accusatory. Focusing on your feelings promotes understanding, while directly blaming someone can be counterproductive as it may make them defensive, hindering constructive communication. Next, the speaking partner expresses their desires. For example, "I desire to feel respected." Then, the speaking partner expresses their boundaries: "My boundary is that if we are having a disagreement, neither of us will raise our voices." To conclude, the speaking partner gets a sacred request. This could be a hug, time alone, a massage, or some other act of love. The listening partner can take a moment to reflect and then try their best to graciously meet this request. Also, only at the very end, it's essential for the listening partner to reflect back the speaking partner's fears, desires, boundaries, and sacred requests like this: "I hear that what I did hurt you, and you desire to feel respected. I will not raise my voice when we disagree. I deeply apologize, and I promise to be more loving. And yes, I'd love to give each other a hug."

### *Learning When to Jump and When to Stay*

It is imperative to surround yourself with people who have similar values, an openness to learn, a heart for growth, and overflow with gratitude. Otherwise, it's like cooking a soup with beautiful organic vegetables but adding pesticide-ridden spices and a broth full of hormones. Toxicity in relationships doesn't happen overnight. If you place a frog in a pot of hot water and gradually heat it up, the frog will adjust to survive and cope. The frog will endure the rising temperature almost until it begins to boil, and then it will die. Don't be like the frog and acclimate yourself to hurtful people or environments, and don't have any kind of relations where toxicity brings you to your breaking point. Relationships of all types are not meant to be endured and coped with; when you engage in them consciously and with clear boundaries, they are how we access deeper levels of true love.

It's natural for people to come and go throughout our life, as they're meant to teach us something. Not everyone is supposed to stay with us throughout time. When we begin vibrating at a different frequency, relationships of all kinds will naturally be drawn to us or repelled. We can love people and still let them go. Fundamentally, people are not meant to be only who we want them to be for us. They are who they are, and we simply get to decide if they are for us or not. When we release attachment to people, places, and things that no longer resonate with us, we open ourselves up to so much more. It is a nuanced process, but you will find that when you start to shift into a new way of being, the people around you that are for you, will understand you, and those who don't, won't. When you shine in your authenticity, you will inspire some people and you will irritate others. All of it is medicine and for the good of all. You are here to walk the unique path that feels good to your heart. Those who resonate with you and share a similar journey will gravitate toward you. Those stuck in their old ways will drift away; it's essential to let them. Remember that everything is here to teach you.

On the other side of releasing old relationships is getting into new ones and committing to those you know. I know it can be scary to let your walls down with new people or forgive someone you love. I've dealt with trauma on every relational level, starting with my father's abandonment and the pain of my mother's neglect. I've been cheated on and have also been unfaithful. I've experienced abusive relationships, been deeply hurt by friends, and have been objectified, assaulted, and abused by multiple men. Also, as a person of color, I am continually given opportunities to heal from and speak to the injustices marginalized peoples and groups have endured.

For many of us, our path has not been convenient or easy. We've had many challenges, asking us to reach deep into ourselves and discover who we are. Doing this and not staying in feelings of blame, shame, anger, or remorse has allowed all traumas and travesties to add to my purpose and support my evolution. This is how I grew. I share my story and these challenges in the hope that you can draw lessons from them and uplift your life. Life is a precious and brief gift. We can't experience every lesson firsthand, which is why sharing our stories is vital. Through them, we can gain wisdom and learn from the experiences of others.

When we have experiences with others that are challenging for reasons we may not understand at the time, they are there to teach us something and help us grow. We must reframe how we view challenges because everything, and I truly mean everything, can be alchemized as an opportunity for growth. Through a combination of resilience and tenderness, I have cultivated gratitude for all of my relations and what they've shown me. So, go as slowly as you need and tune in to your intuition, because there are people with unconscious behaviors or ill intentions. When I haven't listened to the nudges in my heart or the intuitive feelings that tell me something isn't right, I have had to heal from boundaries crossed and harm done. Listen when your intuition says, "Tread carefully," or sometimes even, "Hell no," to a person, place, or thing. Feel, notice, and take action on what your body and soul intelligence is trying to communicate with you.

### *Be in Right Relation in All Your Relations*

I've been able to find deep healing through cultivating sisterhood with those who see me for who I truly am. I also have found brothers who are safe, present, and respect my boundaries. These friendships have been cultivated over years, and for most, there was a knowing that they were people meant for me on a soul level. It wasn't always like this for me. It took time and letting go of old friendships and acquaintances to make space for those who resonated with me on a deeper level. Being in a community, making new friends, and creating relationships may sometimes be challenging as you shed the past and experience change, yet it's soul-fulfilling when you find people who want to evolve alongside you.

Also, I am beyond grateful for the elders, healers, guides, and therapists who have supported me throughout my life. It is important for us to give and receive support from elders and keepers of Indigenous teachings since we have been disconnected from this wisdom. There are many beautiful guides who still practice the ways of their Ancestors, and it is wise to seek them out for your own reclamation and remembrance. It is when we work with guides that we can be held and see the things we wish to bring into the light—learning to acknowledge, feel, and heal, deciding what to carry forward and what to leave behind. Indigenous guides can support us in learning more about our heritage, culture, and traditions. Healers, therapists, mentors, and bodyworkers are also essential allies to cultivate relationships with, as they will show us what we are unaware of and uncover what we haven't been able to work through on our own.

The elders have medicine for us, and the wisdom keepers have beautiful teachings that they pass down for our growth. Yet, it is our responsibility to find what deeply resonates with us and what doesn't. We do not have to take all teachings into the present or continue traditions that we do not feel called to continue. Blind adherence to tradition is also known as dogma. We are being asked to create a new paradigm, as we shift out of disconnection and fear and into connected and faithful ways of being. This means that we are the bridge from the wise ways of our Ancestors to our present life. Since we have such few examples of the quality relationships we wish to see in the world, it's our responsibility to be it.

Remember, guidance isn't solely derived from human teachings. It also comes from your inner knowing, intuition, the energy you possess, and by living a life with a pure and humble heart. The wisdom you seek is already within and all around you. You simply must remember who you truly are and what part you play in harmony with the whole. Discover this and you'll find deep gratitude for all your relationships.

### *Embodiment Practice: The Naming Exercise*

Having clear boundaries is essential to having healthy relationships. When you pay a therapist, that energetic exchange sets clear guidelines in place that you are there for a service. When you work with a healer or mentor, it's obvious that you are coming to them to learn. We have our own homes, our clothes serve as coverings, and even our skin is a boundary, keeping us intact and whole. However, when we experience trauma and our field is penetrated without our consent, this blurs our boundaries and creates ties with painful events or hurtful people. This practice can be used to create a healthy sense of separation from that which no longer serves you.

This Embodiment Practice is called the Naming Exercise. This can be used if you're in a romantic relationship or not, or even to visualize and "call in" a future partner. You can use this toward someone who hurt or abused you, and also to increase healthy magnetism and attraction in your loving relationships. It's one of the most powerful practices for deep healing, claiming your sovereignty, and setting boundaries. This practice is like magic, and it works wonders.

For example, Syris used this practice to release any energy he still carried from a family member who caused him great distress as a child. They did not have a close relationship for their entire lives because of it. But once Syris began doing the Naming Exercise as a part of his daily rituals, they "randomly" called him! His brother wanted to build a closer relationship and acknowledge anything that needed to be resolved from the past so they could have a closer relationship going forward. Just a couple of months later, Syris was one of the first to know when his brother's wife became pregnant.

The Naming Exercise: Find a quiet place where you feel safe and will not be interrupted. You can wear noise canceling headphones (without music), go into a room with the door closed, and do whatever you need to feel comfortable in your own space. Preferably stay standing with your hands comfortably beside you and palms open, facing outward. Take a few slow, deep nasal breaths to fully settle into the space and moment. When you are ready, close your eyes.

Then, call into your mind's eye someone who you feel a strong connection with. This connection can feel healthy if it's someone you love and feel safe with, or it can be someone who hurt you. Regardless of the type of bond you have with them, begin the Naming Exercise by identifying something about your physical self. For example, "My name is Sabrina." Then say, "Your name is ______." Continue to identify physical characteristics that differentiate you from that person. "I have hazel eyes. You have blue eyes." "I am five feet four inches tall. You are over six feet tall." "I have thick black hair. You have wavy blonde hair." Try to keep the things that you use to differentiate yourself from them without emotional charge. Keep them factual and obvious. Keep them based on the attributes that are different from you.

If you find that strong emotions arise during this process, allow them to be felt. You must feel it to heal it, and there's no other time but the present to do so. You can use the Embodiment Practice you learned in Chapter 1 to come back into the space you are in. Give yourself an embrace, and you can even use a mantra from Chapter 2 to help remind you what is true. Then, return to naming things about yourself and them like, "My ears are pierced. Your ears are not."

As you continue holding this person in your mind's eye, naming what makes you, you, and them, them, do so until you see this person as completely separate from you. Once you feel yourself as clearly different from them, use the power of gratitude to transform the relationship. You could experience difficult emotions like resentment, hurt, or sadness. You could also have pleasant feelings of love, familiarity, or comfortability. Regardless of what you feel about this person, speak the following words or something similar that's true for you: "Thank you for what your actions have shown me. All things that you gave me are now returned to you. All that once energetically bound us together is now untied. Thank you, maltyox." Turn your palms inward to yourself, or you can bring them up to your heart. Feel, see, imagine, or visualize that anything of theirs, any energy, memories, past residue, or previous attachments are completely given back to them, and your energy is yours and yours alone.

If you are in a relationship, you can use this practice to increase polarity and magnetism with your partner. Or, if the relationship you're in has caused you pain, this process can help you let go of other people's energy and take back your own energetic space. The key is that this process is based on obvious physical differences to create the clear sense of separation as the foundation. Remember, you now have tools to feel your emotions if they begin to influence how you try and create this healthy sense of separation and sovereignty.

### *Dive Even Deeper . . .*

I invite you to join The United Collective as well as find a community near you that resonates with who you truly are and who you wish to become more like. By doing so, you will find people who align with your values. This can be via in-person activities, virtual communities, online courses, activist groups, or community outreach programs. You can follow @theunitedcollective_ on Instagram to stay updated on future events and connect with a loving community.

CHAPTER 5:

# You Are Always Guided

*"Walking, I am listening to a deeper way.*
*Suddenly, all my Ancestors are behind me.*
*Be still, they say. Watch and listen.*
*You are the result of the love of thousands."*

— LINDA HOGAN

We are all native to this planet with a shared legacy but come from an unknown origin. However, origin myths tell the same basic story. Earth was inhabited by an advanced species as well as hunter-gatherer tribes across the entire planet. Then, a cataclysm of asteroids showered the planet, and great floods followed. After this event, which was so massive it's difficult to even comprehend, myths tell us that great teachers arrived by sea to help the hunter-gatherers around the globe to repopulate the Earth, create civilization, and develop culture.

Carlos Barrios, a famous Mayan elder, shares in *The Book of Destiny* "Accurate accounts of the Maya's origin and arrival on this continent can be found, however, in what are known as the sacred books. The stories sound repetitive or confused at times, but we must remember that the (Mayan) language used at that time is difficult to translate for today's reader." In the Mayan myth, the Feathered Serpent Q'uq'umatz, also known as Quetzalcoatl or Kukulkan, is a mythical culture hero that almost all Mesoamerican peoples claim descent. He came to the hunter-gatherers to form a civilization that honored the Earth and Cosmos. He symbolizes the meeting of the earthly, represented by the snake, and the heavenly, shown by the feathers. This blend makes him a convergence of both land and sky, symbolizing the balance of opposites and connecting both realms. As Carlos Barrios wrote, "Using both cosmic and terrestrial influences, the Maya found a path that follows the Natural Order based on a respect for Mother Nature. Such respect can be summarized in a single word: *harmony*."

The Maya, along with Ancestors from all parts of the world, honored this cataclysmic shift of the planet due to asteroids raining down from the heavens by building temples, mostly pyramid structures, to serve as reminders and a bridge between the Cosmos and the planet. All of the large pyramids and ancient civilizations we see like the Olmecs, Maya, Incan, and others in Southeast Asia, Mesopotamia, North America, and many others, are all unique yet inherently connected. They built these sacred structures to align with the sun, with the solstices, equinoxes, and stars, remembering these defining cosmic occasions via ceremonies. They also created art to commemorate the sole most important event in our collective history, as seen on pillars found at sites like Göbekli Tepe. Now, these key moments in our collective history have been widely forgotten as well as systematically distorted by mainstream historians and archaeologists. We are a forgetful species and need reminding before we completely lose harmony within ourselves, in all our relations, with our Ancestors, the planet, and the Cosmos.

### *Your Ancestors Hold the Keys*

Everyone who's alive today descended from Ancestors who survived this global asteroidal catastrophe, as well as other natural disasters, wars, famine, and diseases. Regardless of whether you come from Mesoamerican, African, Asian, European, Native American, Middle Eastern, or mixed descent, we all share a lineage of those who overcame all odds to remain alive and continue their legacy through us. Unfortunately, many of us have not been taught about our lineages or have had elders or kin that helped us remember the truth of our past.

After surviving unimaginable events and building harmonious civilizations, colonization forced my ancient Mesoamerican Ancestors to abandon their wise traditions. Over time, their descendants took on the culture, religion, and traditions of their oppressors, causing them to forget who they were and where they truly came from. They lost their native tongue, oral histories, traditions, and practices. They were forced to assimilate and fit in with tyrannical, manufactured societies being built around them. For many Ancestors, they had to adapt or they'd be killed. To this day, people of Native descent continue to be forced to conform to limit mistreatment, systemic abuse, suppression, and marginalization.

Our Ancestors were forced to give up their ways and adopt the religions, beliefs, and customs of their oppressors. They were treated as less than human because of their traditions; therefore, most Natives completely abandoned their cultural practices. The adoption of Catholicism, Evangelism, and other denominations of Christianity quickened the erosion of many Indigenous practices. However, these traditions are being revived today through wisdom keepers. Also, people can access this wisdom via dreams, past-life recollections, plant medicine ceremonies, and other altered states of consciousness. The destruction of sacred codices, people being burnt at the stake, slavery, and indentured servitude led to an erasure of Indigenous communities. Western culture, while having many beautiful attributes, caused traumatic disruptions that clearly still affect us today. Due to these horrific events, many descendants of Indigenous lineages have lost touch with their innate strength and the magic of their ancestry.

Our wise Ancestors knew the power of remaining connected to all things. These Ancestors were in tune with the cycles of Earth and the Cosmos. They possessed a powerful communion with the elements, the seen and unseen worlds, and the ever-present magic of life. They honored the heavens as home of the Divine Father and the planet as their first Mother. Her abundant gifts and majesty were revered as sacred, and the temples they built mimicked her grandeur and natural beauty. They were built in alignment with the heavens above, serving as sites to bridge heaven and Earth. In the K'iche Mayan tradition, they call Earth, Heart of the Earth, or "R'ukux Uleu," and God or the Universe, Heart of the Sky, or "R'ukux Kaj." The planet, your body, and these temples are all different iterations of the same thing—vessels that are reflections of, and home to, the Divine.

Thankfully, the ancient ways of these Ancestors have not been entirely destroyed. There are some Maya who have kept their traditions alive through oral teachings. We know some of their history and myths through the codices that were spared. However, only four codices survived being burned by colonizers and Catholic priests. The other ancient texts and teachings were hidden by Mayan elders who retreated into the jungles, likely to never be found or known to the Western world.

If you dive deeply into ancient Mayan history, you will find that these Ancestors were brilliant mathematicians, scientists, and astrologers, to a level that's difficult to fully understand. If you descend from a Mayan lineage, this wisdom lives within you. If you have other genetics, you can learn these teachings from Mayan elders while doing the research to find what remains from your own Indigenous lineages. Having a mentor is essential to support you in your process of coming into full harmony.

In time, you and I will become the Ancestors that our descendants can learn from for support and guidance. In order to be a wise and supportive Ancestor, we must first become balanced within ourselves. If any individual is not aligned within themself, then that's how destructive patterns are perpetuated. When you are not in harmony, you are not in integrity. Any disease, distress, or difficulty you have is a result of living out the destructive patterns that you and your lineage have continued to repeat. Thankfully, you are reading this book because you are here to be the pattern interrupter—the cycle breaker—that can heal, shift, and liberate your lineage.

It is up to us to choose which Ancestors we wish to connect with. Not all are healed or unconditionally loving. Some energies will try to continue living through us, creating deep unconscious behaviors where we don't feel in control of our own lives. We likely do not even know the names of those who impact us now, reaching further back than just our immediate relatives. Thus, we must not lose ourselves by being an empty vessel where unsupportive energies can try to live through us. This is why I continually call in my unconditionally loving Ancestors, and I invite you to do the same.

These wise Ancestors are calling you to heal your bloodline and draw support from the most powerful forces, for there is something to be learned from everything and everyone that came before you. You can access ancient wisdom by calling upon your loving Ancestors, or by working with dreams, meditations, plants, spirit guides, angels, or forces of goodness that operate within other dimensions. We simply have to make the choice to become still, set a heart-centered intention, and listen to whatever messages and guidance comes through. There is deep, ancient wisdom that is waiting to be rediscovered.

I often imagine the era when we honored our differences, reaching even further back to also feel into how we all share a common, albeit specifically unknown, origin. Whenever I walk through museums and sites of ancient ruins like Monte Albán in Oaxaca, Mexico, or Iximche in the highlands of Guatemala, I feel a warmth of remembrance in my blood. I also see the devastation and continued glorification of Catholicism, which then makes my blood boil, saddened that instead of curiosity and collaboration, my Ancestors were massacred.

We are currently living in an era with a tremendous variety of culture, customs, creativity, and access to history, technology, and information. There is so much to be learned from our differences and even more beauty that awaits by claiming our true united history—a history that reaches far beyond our presently recorded understanding. To do so threatens and destabilizes Westernized ways of thinking. To do so is wild and wonderfully courageous, and it will enrich your life. When you remember your roots, the storms can come, the winds will blow, the Earth may tremble, and the fires will blaze, but you'll have all that you need to keep diving deeper into the richness of who you truly are.

As Terence McKenna said, "Nature loves courage. You make the commitment and Nature will respond to that commitment by removing impossible obstacles. Dream the impossible dream and the world will not grind you under; it will lift you up. This is the trick. This is what all these teachers and philosophers who really counted, who really touched alchemical gold, this is what they understood. This is the shamanic dance in the waterfall. This is how magic is done. By hurling yourself into the abyss and discovering it is a feather bed."

### *You Are the Living Answer to Your Ancestors' Prayers*

We can only know true light by going through dark times. This doesn't mean that light is better than darkness. Rather, greater is the light that emerges from darkness. The shadow of harmful, often unconscious, behaviors stem from the unhealed parts of ourselves handed down by our family, surroundings, community, and culture. Whether you descend from Indigenous roots, colonial Ancestors, or are of mixed heritage, your genes carry a deep darkness. This darkness might be ignored, feared, or perhaps you're unsure of how to address it. Yet it's your soul's sacred mission to transform this darkness into light and bring more beauty into the world.

We are meant to learn from and about our past. The best place to learn about ourselves is to explore what did or did not support us during our childhood. We cannot change who our Ancestors are or their actions, but we can choose how we go forward. By releasing them of our expectations, we take back our power and know that it's our sacred responsibility to become who we need for ourselves. You get to be the person now that your younger self would have felt safe with. Doing this, you will reparent yourself. This allows you to let go of expectations from everyone outside of you. When you let go of needing your parents to be someone they weren't, you begin to accept what is, which is reality. Wanting them or your past to be different only causes suffering.

At the deepest root, we must be grateful to our parents for bringing us into this world so that we can experience the fullness of life as a human. Anything else they've provided is a bonus. If there is a part of you that is not grateful for them giving you life, which is truly their only role for you, then you are giving away your power. You do not need to overextend that gratitude to compensate for any troublesome aspects of their character. Simply the act of feeling grateful to them for giving you life allows you to give and receive gratitude at the deepest roots of who you are. Your opportunity to be alive is the greatest gift of all, even though human life is full of challenges.

However, many of us, especially marginalized folk, have inherited generational trauma, systemic suppression, and trickle-down impacts of colonization, slavery, and harmful forms of patriarchy. We must first inform ourselves and each other about these travesties and how they still impact our day-to-day life. We must share our stories. Trauma and abuse are perpetrated behind a veil of ignorance and staying silent. It is up to each one of us to bring things to light and emerge from the darkness of our past, standing up for our entire lineage and becoming who we truly are.

Any resentment of the past will create a fear of the future. Living unhealed, unconscious, or ignorant about the past or future takes us out of the present moment. All things happen only in the present moment, so this moment, and in each recurring moment, is where you get to decide that you are the one to heal yourself, for yourself and for your entire lineage. Doing this, you will learn to make peace with what has happened so you can create a better future. This does not mean you condone your predecessors' hurtful actions, patterns, and behaviors, but you must accept that you cannot change who they are or have been. You hold power over your own inner world and no one else's. You have the infinite potential to change yourself, which is more than enough to create a better world for us all.

You have the endless support of countless unconditionally loving Ancestors who want to see you thrive. Since you are alive, here and now, able-bodied and with a heart of goodness, you can become the living dream of what your Ancestors hoped was possible.

### *A Peek into My Lineage*

As a woman of mixed Indigenous descent, I grew up feeling separate, different, and misunderstood because of oppression, marginalization, and racism. I am also healthy and able-bodied, which has afforded me great privilege. I have walked in both worlds. I have felt less than and better than. I have felt it all, because I am it all. I have blood made up of both the victim and the perpetrator, the colonized and the colonizer. Forgetfulness and remembrance run through my veins.

Like most first-, second-, or third-generation immigrants, I was completely severed from my roots. For most of my life, I had no sense of connection to my Indigenous background because my mother and grandmother never talked about their Native cultures, and my father wasn't around while I was growing up. I am mixed, and known as a mestizo. This is a term used in Mesoamerica to describe people of mixed European and Indigenous American descent. The word itself originates from the Latin *mixticius*, meaning "mixed," yet historically, this phrase has been and can be negatively used to disconnect people from identifying with their Indigenous roots. My mother is a first generation Mexican-American. My maternal grandma, who was also my primary caregiver for many years, was native to Juárez, Mexico, so I have Aztecan and Mayan Ancestors from her lineage. My maternal grandfather is a mix of European descent and is from Pennsylvania, in the USA. My father was from Guatemala. When he was around five years old, he fled to the United States with his mother and brothers due to the Guatemalan Civil War. My father was a mestizo, too, being part Maya, and somewhere down the line, he gained Spanish roots.

My parents met in California while in high school, conceiving me just before my father got involved with drugs and gangs. One of my first memories included him. I was about three, and he came for a visit. Together with my mother, we went to a drive-in movie. That would be the last time I saw him until I turned 13. He was in and out of my life from the age of 13 until I was 18. I only met him a handful of times, but he sent me encouraging letters throughout that time, which kept me hopeful for a future connection. But after he tragically passed away, I closed myself off from anything to do with him, which severed me from my roots.

During my childhood I would sometimes join my grandma and mother when they'd go to the Catholic church, and I experienced Christian churches with childhood friends. Spirit undeniably moves through all expressions of life, but these religious rituals didn't feel natural to me. I didn't know it at the time, but the purity of my heart, the Native wisdom that flows through my blood, and the pre-colonial traditions embedded in my DNA knew what I was experiencing wasn't meant for me.

Most of my family members unconsciously perpetuated cycles of abuse, alcoholism, religious dogma, and other inherited products of patriarchy and colonization. Since I experienced trauma in my households, I was naturally closed off to relating with my family. I would attend gatherings, but there was an underlying sense of discomfort and dread that kept me feeling separate and misunderstood. For example, I might have been at a birthday party or quinceañera, but I don't remember feeling fully safe or free to enjoy myself. I was hypervigilant, especially around my family.

I am aware that many people have and maintain a strong connection to their biological family and the culture they're born into. Especially among all Latin American cultures, family is at the core. You're taught to always be there for your family, even if that means disregarding your boundaries. While being close-knit has its advantages, the fact remains that blindly adhering to family and cultural norms can hinder many from connecting with their authentic selves and deepest roots.

Conforming to, going along with, or feeling a deep sense of obligation to post-colonial cultures means that millions of people are living the limited dreams of their colonized Ancestors. Mariachi, fiestas, and other traditions—while they all have their place and time, and do serve as moments of significant connection with loved ones—exist because of Spanish colonization. Additionally, blending Latin culture with the "American Dream" has buried the ancient DNA, wise ways, and innate connectedness that we all have.

In the past, I felt strong dissonance to Latin culture. For years, I felt ashamed for not speaking Spanish. The disapproving looks first came from my family, but even well into adulthood from Latine, Chicane, and Central American communities. Simultaneously, being born and raised in the United States, I also felt ashamed for not being white enough. It seemed to me that wherever I was or whatever I was doing, someone would be there to remind me I was doing it wrong and essentially, that I was wrong. Being of mixed heritage can often feel like navigating a perpetual, challenging tug-of-war. Yet it's a gift to have multiple traditions and cultures contained within our blood. Beyond appearances and heritage, there's a deeper essence that defines us. This unique blend not only enriches our personal experiences but also allows us to bridge gaps, fostering understanding and unity among diverse communities. It empowers us to be ambassadors of harmony, sharing stories from every facet of our lineage and reminding the world of the beauty in diversity.

Once I began living on my own, I started attending fewer family functions. For me, it was easier to leave my past in the past and move toward things that felt new, gave me freedom, but also seemed safer than what I was coming from. Some people express their desire for safety by staying where they're at; I did so by venturing into new opportunities to escape what I was born into. I became friends with people of all backgrounds and dated many types of men, but I felt the safest with white men—because they didn't look like any of my relatives. I dated men of color, but those relationships never lasted. My surroundings reinforced that white men were safer than Brown men. It was societal, too: consider that at that time, everything in the media, whether the news or movies, confirmed that the safe and noble men were like John Smith from Pocahontas, and never the equally handsome Kocoum.

I found it a relief to immerse myself in my partner's life and his traditions rather than speak about or have curiosity of my own. I wanted nothing to do with my Latina, Chicana, or Indigenous roots, not that I even knew anything about my Mayan and Mexica roots at that time. The only things I thought I knew about Mayan or Mexica culture was from the 2006 movie *Apocalypto,* which portrayed Mesoamericans as savages. I also heard that the Maya predicted the "end of the world" in 2012, but then that didn't happen, further delegitimizing my faith or curiosity toward ancient ideas. It was easier to learn about other traditions, since during my childhood and adolescence, I didn't learn one positive thing about my culture. I became fascinated by Asian culture and food, and then, yoga was easy for me to connect with, since there was no personal or generational trauma involved with it.

Those of mixed descent have had excessive racist and discriminatory programming, reaching back many generations and continuing now. For example, Ricardo Cajas, Guatemala's former presidential commissioner on racism, stated that *Apocalypto* set back understanding of the Mayan people by 50 years, comparing its impact to that of the negative images of Native Americans in movies from the 1950s. Cajas said, "It shows the Mayans as barbarous, murderous people that can only be saved by the arrival of the Spanish."

Ignacio Ochoa boldly stated that this film perpetuated "an offensive and racist notion that Mayan people were brutal to one another [ . . . ] and thus deserved rescue."

Such portrayals of Indigenous cultures perpetuate harmful stereotypes, leading marginalized communities, people of color, and those with Native heritage to unconsciously distance themselves from their roots. However, when we uncover the truth about our Ancestors and recognize their achievements, our perspective shifts. The Mayan civilization, for example, was advanced in numerous areas. They had a complex hieroglyphic writing system, were adept at mathematics and astronomy, and had a calendar system more accurate than the Julian calendar used in Europe. Their architectural feats, such as complex highways and roads, as well as pyramids at Tikal and Palenque, demonstrate their engineering skills. In agriculture, they pioneered techniques like terracing, biochar, and crop rotation, enabling them to sustain large populations in challenging environments. When we realize that they were primarily peaceful, deeply connected to Earth and the Cosmos, and lived in harmony with the rhythms of nature, we come to understand the profound wisdom and beauty our Ancestors possessed. It's a privilege to be alive at this time, where we have the opportunity to rediscover and honor the powerful legacy of our forebears.

Those of us who have mixed lineage hold the gift of multiple traditions and dynamic genetics. We are privileged to be a bridge between the Native and the Westernized. We have the sacred responsibility to be the embodiment of love as we right the wrongs of the past, honor our Indigenous kin, share our wise ways, and choose how we live going forward. Speaking English and Spanish, both languages of colonizers, gives us access to speak to more hearts, and our mixed blood gives us the ability to have compassion for all peoples. Present generations can change how things have been done before us and usher in a new way of being by shining light on the fear, separation, capitalism, and neo-colonization that continues to destroy this world and not give equitable opportunity to marginalized peoples. Your life can be an example of what it looks like to awaken to your ancestral power, remember your roots, and live life in gratitude!

It wasn't until I discovered Mayan ceremonial cacao in 2016 that I learned something positive, beautiful, or empowering about my Ancestors. Mayan cacao is a sacred plant medicine that reconnected me to my heart, to my lineage, and to my Ancestors. As soon as the teacher told me that the Maya people from Guatemala made the cacao we were drinking, I reclaimed a buried part of myself. I opened up to the guidance of my Ancestors and immediately knew I was meant to work with this plant for my own healing and the healing of the world. It was a calling, a knowing that this was something significant for me, my lineage, and many others.

Cacao was the initial bridge that connected me back to my Ancestors and my Native roots, and your bridge may be something entirely different. Indigenous traditions are simple and intuitive. If something resonates, trust that call. It's your soul reconnecting with ancient truths. There may be another ancestral plant that calls to you, or you may possibly feel connected to your roots via a drum, tree, location, or from remembering a dream, vision, or magical experience you've had. Don't be afraid to simply begin, to look silly, or to feel weird within yourself by doing something out of the ordinary. Whatever calls to you is perfect to get you started on the path of reconnecting with your roots.

Regardless of your lineage as revealed by tests like 23andMe or AncestryDNA, regardless of your physical appearance, skin color, eye shade, or the language you speak, assimilation and displacement cannot erase your intrinsic Indigenous identity. Your essence is firmly rooted in the ancient ways of the Indigenous. As you journey to reconnect with your origins, you'll find the insights of the ancient Ancestors resonating more deeply with you than perhaps even the kin you've known in this life.

### *Re-Indigenizing*

"Decolonization" is the process of deprogramming from colonial mindset. However, this focuses on colonization rather than placing Indigenous peoples' journey of reclaiming, reconnecting, and remembering as the focus of the process. We aim to see through our own lens, from our perspective. Rather than continuing to base our identity on decolonization, we must prioritize "re-Indigenization." This involves actively seeking to bond with our ancestral knowledge and traditions. It's about more than just dismantling old frameworks; it's about reviving and celebrating our innate, profound ways. Both processes, regardless of your specific ancestry, are vital, be it for direct ancestral healing or supportive allyship.

While we are all one human race, it's essential to respect distinctive Indigenous cultures, customs, and practices. There is a fine line between cultural appreciation and cultural appropriation. Cultural appropriation is harmful to Indigenous people because it perpetuates taking from them without reciprocity, care, honor, or respect. There has not been enough acknowledgment, reconciliation, or collective healing for Indigenous people, so appropriation still exists. It's essential to have a deep understanding that Indigenous people have and continue to be harmed. Taking or using their practices without their permission and not empathizing with their hardships perpetuates colonization. By not acknowledging and understanding the depth of their experiences, we inadvertently silence their voices and minimize their struggles, further deepening the divide and perpetuating injustices.

It's important for us to be able to put ourselves in others' experiences and feel for those who've had different upbringings and experiences. This includes a deep honoring of the inequalities and injustices that People of Color experience. We cannot skip over the messy parts when coming back into wholeness. The dark and difficult history of colonization and erasure of Indigenous peoples have been ignored for too long. We must acknowledge the ways in which we have harmed or been harmed in direct and indirect ways. Also, we must acknowledge the ways in which we have perpetuated or been complicit in creating forms of separation as well. We must realize how we have been privileged or experienced power imbalances in our environments. Most importantly, we must nurture our hearts and address the pain we and our Ancestors endured, ensuring that these deep wounds heal and aren't carried forward to future generations.

Indigenous peoples need allies and to be uplifted after being demonized and victimized for so long. Since most Native peoples are fundamentally nonviolent, they are easy to take from. They live in reciprocity with the planet and others, seeking to collaborate, not compete. They deserve to be appreciated; therefore we must honor, respect, and care for Native people and their practices. This is an invitation for you to connect with and collaborate with those who are Indigenous, but to do so with humility. If it's your own culture that you want to connect with, come to learn with an open and pure heart. Honor the wisdom keepers that have kept the traditions alive against all odds and know that your Indigenous Ancestors have been waiting for you to reclaim your birthright.

We must re-Indigenize ourselves in honor of the Ancestors who were not allowed to be themselves, practice their customs, or speak their truth. When we know who we are and where we come from, we can heal from any harm caused and live out our purpose. By reclaiming our roots, we can trace our lineage back to find that we are all connected in the web of life. When we deeply know our truth and our whole selves, we can feel how we belong here and deserve to live beauty-filled lives.

If you have felt any resistance or can imagine how others would be resistant to reclaiming what has been taken, know that it can take time to access your innately magical and wise ways after so much trauma from the not-so-distant past. The way we move through this resistance is to acknowledge that we have felt ignored and have in turn ignored our connection to our roots. Then, we must feel compassion for ourselves and for the journey our Ancestors have been on. You have the courage encoded in your DNA to hold all things, especially yourself, gently and tenderly.

### *More Than Enough*

There are still many Indigenous people who do not feel safe to practice their ancestral ways; and in some parts of the Americas, it still isn't safe. Colonial programming has indoctrinated many Indigenous people to live a dogmatic Christian, Evangelical, or Catholic way of life. In many parts of Guatemala, there are Evangelicals who are so disconnected from their roots, they superstitiously believe that Indigenous ways are evil. As recently as 2020, a Mayan spiritual guide in Chimay, Guatemala, was burned at the stake by a mob; they were upset because someone who had sought help from the healer had passed away. These people show the most extreme residual impact of colonization.

However, these neo-colonial ways of thinking are how many of our relatives, parents, or grandparents still believe and act today, even if they don't show it directly. It is sadly ironic that people of Indigenous descent have been conditioned to be fearful of the very thing that could give them freedom and power. Personally, I believe the reason it's so extreme in Guatemala is because the civil war there only ended in the 1990s, the decade after I was born. Over 626 massacre sites have been found, and over 250,000 Guatemalans were massacred, most of them being Indigenous Maya. This has affected the Mayan population tremendously, yet Guatemala still has the most Mayan people per capita.

These events have left an enduring negative impact on many Mayan people's physical, mental, and spiritual health. "The killing of so many Mayans badly damaged their transmission of oral history and traditional knowledge, such as the use of local plants as medicines and traditional healthcare and their own language and cultural practices. There was also a land dimension to the genocide, where people were forcibly displaced to make way for large-scale farming, mining, and hydroelectric programs," writes Luke Moffett in his article published in *The Conversation*.

Tragedies like these are what have kept many Mayan people disempowered. That story ends when we see that it is not only safe to reclaim our Indigenous roots, but it is critical for our healing. It is essential to reclaim the parts of ourselves that have been shunned and persecuted. For you to be who you're meant to be in the world, you must know the truth of who you are and where you come from. When we integrate this remembrance into our lives, we can heal our entire future lineage, live in alignment with our truth, and activate our life's purpose.

I want every person who has Ancestors that were Native to the Americas to contemplate the fact that their language was not Spanish. This is a colonizing language. Your Indigenous lineage's languages may be Nahuatl, K'iche, Otomanguean, Mixe-Zoque, Totonacan, Uto-Aztecan, Chibchan, Quechua, Aymara, Tupí-Guaraní, Mapuche, or another. Language is very important, for it is what we use to pass on stories, information, myths, and remembrance. Knowing the true word of something connects you to the essence of that thing. That is why when we use ancient words, it feels different. Saying *maltyox* invokes a different energy and more powerful frequency than just saying thank you. Learning more about Indigenous languages is a direct access point to keeping the wisdom of your Ancestors alive.

We all take different paths to reclaiming our roots. Remember that feeling worthy to reclaim your truth and wisdom can sometimes feel challenging in the beginning. This is because many of our Ancestors were shamed, and we can still carry shame within us. It's not easy to move through the impacts of forced indoctrination and assimilation. It can be easier to connect with other cultures' practices because they don't carry generational trauma for us. As I mentioned previously, in the beginning of my healing journey, it was much easier for me when I was learning about yogic traditions rather than Mayan traditions. It takes intentional effort to decolonize and re-Indigenize ourselves so that we can deepen our roots. Re-Indigenizing our lives is reclamation work. We are reclaiming the parts of ourselves that have been cast aside, forgotten, and oppressed for too long so that we can feel our wholeness and enoughness.

There is a distortion that has been programmed into BIPOC, Latine, Chicane, Indigenous, and even allies of these groups. We have likely felt ashamed of our roots or not good enough to claim this part of ourselves. I share this wisdom so you can take what resonates and live in harmony with your inner and outer worlds like your wise Ancestors did. Of course, not all Ancestors were perfect, and not all Indigenous teachings are perfect either.

It's crucial to remain heart-centered, physically grounded, and yet receptive to mentors on our journey. No elder or teaching should override our intuition, nor should we think one person or group holds all the answers. When gaps appear in understanding and we're told "that's just the way things are" without room for inquiry or evolution, that's when beliefs turn dogmatic. That represents an outdated paradigm. We are here to create a new reality that respects both our history and the promise of a bright future. This vision recognizes our innate wisdom and intuition, and it seeks a dance between masculine and feminine energies, between Earth and the Cosmos, and between the Divine and the human experience. We are all experiencing a collective awakening to a more harmonious, equitable, and sustainable way of life, where humanity and the planet thrive in a reciprocal relationship.

I want every person with Indigenous roots to know that you are not less than, you are not broken, and you are more powerful than you have ever imagined. Healing is possible by getting still enough to listen to the magic within the unseen worlds, within nature, through your own inner wisdom, and through your dreams and visions. When you become quiet, purge yourself from neocolonialism, and re-Indigenize yourself, coming home to yourself is inevitable. You must move out of suppression, through separation, and into true connection to activate the wisdom that's been lying dormant within your bones. Your living body holds both the light and dark and is medicine for your evolution. This life is a journey—a walk back home to yourself, not a marathon to be won.

### *Conclusion*

Ancestral connections are not limited to those with whom we share a biological link. They also include individuals with whom we have a profound spiritual bond. Activities like dancing, singing, and cooking, as well as practices like ritual, prayer, and meditation, are channels through which we can forge these connections. The wisdom of our Ancestors may have been buried, but the strength of our roots remains unbroken. This resilience prepares us to unearth our inherent power and magic, especially at this pivotal time in the world. Ancestral work serves as a reminder that we belong and that a supportive community is always there for us to call upon.

Your Ancestors are more than just the humans that came before you, but also includes the wisest shamans, midwives, healers, warriors, astrologers, and artists, reaching all the way back to the elements of fire, wind, earth, and water, for this is what you are made of. Your Ancestors include the rivers, rocks, and soils, all of which descend from stardust. Your body is made up of recycled hawk feathers, jaguar claws, butterfly wings, and bear fur. All of it is in you. You have the same elements that make up the vast ocean within your blood. The same minerals, like calcium, that form sand are in your bones.

Your ancestry is what can be called forth out of the Great Mystery to remind you of your connection to all things. By recognizing the vastness of your ancestry, you tap into elemental magic that affirms you are a living, breathing embodiment of all that has come before you. Engaging with the elements, you form a bridge to the wisdom of your Ancestors, hearing them in the crackle of fire, seeing them in the flow of water, feeling them in the wind, and walking with them on Earth.

We are not alone in the work we do to heal ourselves. When you open yourself up to the loving Ancestors, you can allow them to guide you, protect you, and support your healing. This can be as simple as using your voice to call upon them. Sometimes the most profound things are truly the simplest that have just been forgotten. Even if you're skeptical at first, this work has evidence-backed benefits for mental health. By engaging with your Ancestors, you not only facilitate your own healing but also contribute to the collective well-being of both living and deceased relatives.

It's your responsibility to carry forward the strengths and address the weaknesses you've inherited, shaping a better future not only for yourself but also for the generations that will follow. In doing so, you fulfill the hopes and prayers of your Ancestors, ultimately working to benefit those who will come after you. This is how we heal intergenerational trauma; this is how we become the cycle breakers and the ones the Ancestors have been waiting for.

We are not bound to repeat history or to adhere rigidly to the practices of those who came before us. Rather, we are meant to glean wisdom from the past, selecting the parts that will propel us toward a healthy and hopeful future while letting go of what no longer serves us. In this light, I call upon the untainted wisdom and magic of your Ancestors—those who existed before colonization forced them to alter their way of life—to guide and support you.

### *Embodiment Practice: Ancestral Meditation*

It is powerful to have a devotional practice, also known as a ritual, that keeps your body, mind, and soul in alignment. This will keep you open to receive support from your Ancestors and guides. You can receive guidance by asking a question before you sleep, pulling a card from an oracle deck, or meditating. The answers may come through in visualizations, images, thoughts, or sensations. They may not come right when you ask for them to, and you may not consciously realize your question has been answered. Guidance might come through during a walk, during prayer, dancing, cooking, singing, dream space, or even through bodywork. When you are in an open and relaxed state, you can receive messages. Time basking in nature, going into the ocean, meditating with a candle flame, and connecting with the elements is another way you can communicate with your Ancestors. The more you practice listening to and trusting the unseen dimensions, the more you will receive.

This practice is an ancestral meditation. Set the space by cleansing the energy. You can burn blessing herbs like locally grown and sustainably harvested sage, tobacco, palo santo, cedar, sweetgrass, or lavender. Burning these herbs reconnects us with Spirit and the unseen worlds. It purifies the energy around you and brings you into harmony. You can also gather a bundle of cedar or rosemary and sprinkle some Agua de Florida around the space to clear the energy. If you have none of those things to clear the space, use sound from a drum, sound bowl, or your own voice by humming.

Put on some beautiful meditation music with drums, nature sounds, flutes, or whatever feels natural for you to listen to. Have someone read this next part to you or record yourself reading it slowly and play the recording so that you can drop into your body and imagination fully. Make sure to sit up nice and tall, keeping your spine straight, or lie down.

Next, take a few deep breaths, inhaling through the nose and exhaling through the mouth. Do this slowly, presently, and intentionally. In your own time, return to normal breathing. Feeling yourself relax with every breath you take, relaxing into receiving. Open your heart to receive from your Ancestors.

See, feel, or imagine walking yourself through the front door of your home and entering into a meadow that leads to a majestic forest. Feel your feet on the earth, the soft soil and grass between your toes. Feel the breeze gently licking your skin, the sound of the wind whispering sweet greetings. The sun is kissing your face and warming your body. You can hear the birds chirping and singing sweetly.

See yourself walking toward and slowly placing your hands upon an ancient tree. As you do this, you are able to see with your mind's eye, beyond the bark of the tree trunk, into its energetic workings. You see that its roots are intertwined under the soil below you, reaching deep into the darkness. Its branches reach toward the sun high in the sky. In a playful dance with the wind, the roots are grounded, solid, and secure in the soil of the First Mother.

Sit with your back against the tree and ask to receive a most beloved and wise Ancestor to be with you now. Feel, see, or sense this Ancestor before you. Perhaps you visualize someone specific; it could be an animal, a plant, an element, or a memory that comes to you. Sit with them in full presence. Feel their essence without needing to fill the space with words or thoughts. Breathe here for as long as feels natural.

If you feel it is time, ask your Ancestor a question that you have in your heart or simply open to receive their guidance or wisdom. Receive this message through visualization, thoughts, memories, feelings, or emotions. After you feel complete, give thanks for their presence and the gift of life that they have afforded you. Give thanks for their support. Give thanks from the depths of your heart for them and release this vision.

Imagine yourself standing under this tree, giving thanks for it being the bridge between light and dark, earth and sky. In your own time, come back to your home and into the space around you. Wiggle your fingers and toes, and when you are ready, open your eyes. Retrieve your journal to write about your journey and the guidance that was imparted to you. You may continue to receive messages from this Ancestor through your physical world or in your dream space. Stay open, observational, and conversational.

CHAPTER 6:

# Plants Are Our Allies

*"What if you were a teacher but had no voice to speak your knowledge? What if you had no language at all, and yet there was something you needed to say? Wouldn't you dance it? Wouldn't you act it out? Wouldn't your every movement tell the story? In time you would be so eloquent that just to gaze upon you would reveal it all. And so it is with these silent green lives."*

— Robin Wall Kimmerer

Plants are magical, intelligent, and ancient allies that exist to support our growth, healing, and evolution. Each plant is a world unto itself, a microcosm we collectively barely understand. Like all things, there is depth and richness within plants that Indigenous people have known and honored. Most Native cultures lived in or around jungles, rainforests, and luscious landscapes, surrounded by fruits, herbs, and medicines many of us can only attempt to imagine. Others who lived near deserts also were in deep communion with the wisdom of the plants and animals they cohabited with.

The plants are allies for our life's journey. When we ingest plants, they provide us essential nutrients, while others open our inner eyes to discover deeper truths than what is available to us in our normal state. They shift us, teach us, fuel us, heal us, and they are here for and with us. Living in a state of reciprocity—and ultimately gratitude—for all plants opens us up to receive the gifts of the life-giving vegetation that our planet offers in abundance. They also embody personalities and have characteristics that humans are wise to emulate. Plants hold beauty in their audacity as they shine without apology. It's as if they exist in all their magic and splendor to remind us of how to grow and thrive in our unique way.

For millions of years, humans evolved alongside flora and fauna, which makes plants and animals our kin. There are certain plants that serve as medicines for specific human organs. Even though most of us are disconnected from plants other than having a salad or herbal supplement, without them, humans would not possibly exist. Trees produce roughly 30 percent of all breathable oxygen, and marine plants like plankton produce 50 to 80 percent. What we breathe out, they breathe in.

We can learn so much from trees. The tree is connected to the vast network of life; it is inherently grounded to the Mother and connected with the worlds around, above, and below it. The further the tree's roots grow, the more its branches expand and its leaves reach to the sky. It receives energy and lives because of the light of the sun. In return the tree grows beautifully, shining in its authentic beauty without ever thinking twice if it is taking up too much space. It gives back by giving nutrients to other trees through its connection to the other root systems, supported by mushroom mycelium. It gives us air, nutrients within its abundant fruits, shade underneath its branches, and energetically we can feel its life-giving and loving energy. It gives so much and receives so much, growing and glowing in all of its glory. The tree is grounded, rooted; it flows, it grows, it gives, and it receives. The tree is the embodiment of a reciprocal and grateful existence. The tree is the ultimate metaphor for our own life—living in a balanced, natural, and grounded way.

On every level, and regardless of whether someone knows it or not, we are in a relationship with Nature. We have the privilege to be alive, to be conscious and aware of our environments; and it is our duty to give our deepest gratitude to Mother Nature. May we all remember that it is a privilege to be a steward of this planet and that plants, animals, and all living things are our sisters and brothers.

### *Nature Provides the Ultimate Luxury*

As a teen raised in a low-income household, I developed a craving for luxury. Since I didn't feel cared for, it was easy to perceive that people who lived extravagantly were genuinely happy. Money seemed to be the ultimate solution because I always felt better after my mom would take me to Goodwill, the Swap Meet, or Ross to buy me new things. If money made me feel better, then why not try to get more of it? Or so I thought. While my mother couldn't meet my emotional needs, she showed her love by spending what little money she had on toys and clothing. But at that time, she had a shopping problem, just like my grandmother. They told me that I better work hard so that I could buy lots of stuff too. Instead of spending money as soon as I got it like them, I saved because I desperately wanted to move into my own place.

At 13, I started working as my neighbor's babysitter. I would also shop often, but not so much that it would affect my obsession with saving. My grandfather taught me that saving was important because "you never know when the money would stop coming in." This sense of lack and scarcity around money added more legitimacy to the belief that I needed money to feel safe.

We learn through examples of what we see modeled around us. But since I didn't like what I was around, I looked out into society to provide me with answers. What a mistake that was, but I didn't know any better. My mom, her brothers, and my grandparents have all lived within 30 minutes of each other their entire lives. Still to this day, many of them think that's normal and that I'm the one who's lost.

I wanted freedom, success, and adventure. I worked part-time at various jobs while putting myself through college debt-free, graduating with an associate's degree in social and behavioral health science. I worked in sales for years because my degree didn't help me make money. Eventually, I moved to Los Angeles and worked odd jobs. I was a server, a leasing agent, and then became a real estate agent. While in LA, I lived a luxurious life. I made good money, and the circles I was in allowed me the privilege of dating men who were even more successful than me and would show off to get my attention. Even though I was living the life 13-year-old me dreamed of, I always felt like I was poor, the success wouldn't last, and deep down, I was undeserving of such luxury. It was a sad feeling.

Underneath the glitz and glam, I was a troubled person, but I always had a big smile on my face. It was a scary season of life, yet I stayed busy so I didn't ever have to feel my sadness. I never liked crying in front of anyone for anything, preferring to disassociate and numb myself. Operating this way for years, I inevitably developed many health issues like irritable bowel syndrome, severe acid reflux, and lactose intolerance.

Even though I seemingly had so much, I wasn't able to feel gratitude sustainably, nor did I even know that gratitude was something important to feel. Regardless of what I had, experienced, or was given, I always wanted more. Just like my mother, grandmother, and family that I once so badly wanted to be different from, I was addicted to quick fixes to feel a sense of joy. I was fully reliant on partners, others, and a lifestyle to feel good. My health got worse until I decided I needed to change. Sometimes we don't realize we're in over our heads until we start drowning.

It was only when I hit my rock bottom that I realized that I wanted to live. That is one thing about hitting the bottom: you have no choice but to know that you are coming up. So, when times get tough, you must ask yourself, "What is this here to teach me, and how can it assist me on my come up? How can I transmute, transform, or compost this into fertilizer for my growth and expansion?" I chose to swim to the top, slowly learning how to ride the waves of life, day by day. Yoga helped me to feel safe in my body, and cacao allowed me to dive deeper into feeling my emotions.

It is good medicine to feel our challenging feelings. When we start to feel all of our emotions, we stop seeing them as only positive or negative, and they lose their intense charge. A heavy emotion can perhaps be associated with a feeling of sadness, but that doesn't mean it's something bad. We get to trust in the unfolding of life, grateful for all things. We also get to remember that we mustn't do it all alone. Plants, herbs, mushrooms, animals, walks in nature, sunlight, tending to a garden, fingernails in the dirt, toes on the ground, and hands to the sky; oh, all the things we are supported by!

There is a difference between consuming to fill an inner void versus appreciating comfort and luxury with intention. You will know the difference if you're experiencing gratitude for what you have and actively seek out how to share your abundance with others rather than keeping it all for yourself. You will feel less likely to go shopping unless you truly need something. You will find that quality products are more fulfilling than an excessive quantity. You'll also need much less than you've previously needed. You won't need a dozen shoes or dresses in every different color. You won't need nearly as much makeup or hair tools. You will begin to truly appreciate garments that are comfortable and made sustainably. Essentially, you won't use things to make you feel better about yourself.

When you feel gratitude for yourself and for all things, you will treat life with reverence. You will want to buy quality clothes to honor and adorn your body as a temple. You will want to respect the garment for it providing you comfort and the feeling of luxury. You will honor the life you intake to sustain you, and you will learn to commune with Nature. By remembering that you are interconnected with the living intelligence of the entire Universe, you will know that you are never alone. Nature is always there ready to support you, provide for you, comfort you, and love you.

### *Be an Ally to Your Allies*

It wasn't until I worked with Mayan ceremonial cacao that I realized when we have food in right relation, it is medicine for body, mind, and soul. Cacao is a gentle plant medicine, yet it is profound for heart healing and creating coherence between the body, mind, and soul. Ceremonial cacao means the cacao is produced traditionally and ceremoniously. It is grown organically by Mayan farmers, and then harvested, prepared, roasted, and processed into chocolate with love, thoughtfulness, blessings, and prayers poured into it. From the tree to the drink, it is made with intention. Ceremonial cacao undergoes minimal processing so as to not kill the living enzymes and the healing properties within it, such as antioxidants, phenethylamine (PEA), anandamide, monoamine oxidase inhibitors (MAOIs), minerals, and vitamins.

Unlike our ancient Ancestors who used to eat plants in their whole form, we now eat highly processed foods. This processing removes the essential minerals, nutrients, and vitamins plants naturally have that support our mood and give us sustained health. PEA is called the "love chemical," and is a natural chemical that boosts happiness and feelings of love in the brain. It's the feeling we get when we are around someone we deeply love and are completely absorbed in the moment with them. PEA supports our dopamine levels and keeps us in a positive mood for longer. People with depression, PTSD, and some types of addiction have low levels of PEA. Anandamide is sometimes called the "bliss molecule" because it supports us in feeling mildly euphoric. *Ananda* means "bliss" in Sanskrit, one of the world's oldest languages. MAOIs are enzymes that help to keep us feeling blissed out for longer. The combination of all these is only within cacao in its natural form, making ceremonial cacao good for the body and extraordinarily supportive for our healing.

Cacao is also considered an adaptogen. Adaptogens are types of plants, herbs, mushrooms, or in this case a tree, that help our body manage stress and restore balance after a stressful situation. What makes this group of plant allies special is how they support the other plants around them growing in their natural environment. The cacao tree, just like mushrooms, can communicate with other plants, sending whatever minerals or nutrients they need to thrive. It has the ability to "adapt" to its environment, serving as a master architect by creating a thriving ecosystem.

Mushrooms communicate to trees, plants, and entire ecosystems through tiny threads that spread throughout the soil called mycelium. These mycelial networks are how forests, fields, jungles, and rainforests are fully alive and in constant communication with each other. Therefore, when you eat medicinal mushrooms, or other adaptogens like ashwagandha, ginseng, tulsi/holy basil, cacao, and others, you are able to be supported in stress adaptation, gain essential minerals, and help restore nervous system regulation. Every person is different, so it is important to notice how each herb, plant, food, fruit, or nourishment makes your body feel.

Cacao is also a subtle consciousness-shifting plant, but it is not psychoactive. Other amazing plants in this category are blue lotus, lavender, kanna, and kava. They soothe our minds, open our hearts, relax our nervous system, expand our consciousness, and also assist us in regulating our nervous system. This type of plant works through subtlety and gentleness, allowing us to tap into the magic that is ever-present all around us. They remind us of our interconnection to the living world within the unseen worlds, helping us feel what has been obscured by conditioning.

There exist more intense consciousness-shifting plant medicines like ayahuasca, yagé, psilocybin mushrooms, and iboga. While there is tremendous, beautiful work being done to support people with addictions, depression, PTSD, and many other mental, emotional, and spiritual disturbances, I personally tread very lightly with these plant medicines. From what I have seen, in many ways, psychedelic medicines have become yet another frontier that Western society has colonized. With the resurgence of plant medicine, it has become a tourist attraction in places like Peru, Costa Rica, and other popular destinations for expats.

While it's no laughing matter, many of the original medicine keepers of ayahuasca do laugh or shake their heads when they hear of ceremonies being held in Los Angeles, Brooklyn, or Miami because to purely experience the plant medicine, one must be in the environment where it comes from. Sadly, many people engage in an unhealthy dynamic with intensely psychoactive plant medicines. People give their power away and claim a certain medicine will heal them, heal the world, and "fix" their problems.

In the Wise Woman tradition of folk herbalism, the most fundamental belief is that nobody is ever sick or needs to be fixed. This is yet another product of a mechanistic, masculine-dominant worldview. Rather, someone may be out of alignment, and certain plants, used in certain ways, can support the person regaining their own alignment. This is a subtle but critical shift of perspective to have—one of reciprocity, not reliance. In this way, we seek not only what we can receive, but what we can give in return.

However, if someone remains imbalanced for long enough, has an unhealthy environment, and is dysregulated in body, mind, or spirit, this will manifest as a physical ailment. Fundamentally, illness is not something to be cured. It is a product of something being out of alignment. In the most critical instances, like cancer, nerve damage, diabetes, etc., modern medicine is likely the best route to take so as to not pass away prematurely. Natural medicines, and regarding food as medicine, is essential to prevent major illnesses or regain health after experiencing an illness.

First and foremost, I am an advocate for gentle consciousness-shifting plants that are easy on our nervous system. Only after someone has devoted time to work with a gentle medicine, herb, or plant should they open up to working with more intense plant medicines. Many psychedelic plant medicines have been exploited and are not being shared in integrity. Also, if you're someone who's never worked with Indigenous wisdom, herbalism, or culture, by going straight to some of the most potent medicines they offer, like ayahuasca, you miss out on learning the vast, rich, and incredible wisdom these lineages hold in the simple, subtle, and sacred aspects of their day-to-day living. To go straight to the most intense or seemingly beautiful thing and take it over and over, never pausing long enough to immerse oneself in the majesty of true reverence, gratitude, and reciprocity, is to perpetuate exactly what the colonizers did and is unfortunately how many people still live today.

If or when you do experience a higher-intensity consciousness-shifting plant medicine, which I do think would be beneficial to many people, know that you will be in one of the most vulnerable states of your life. It's a full process of metaphorical death and rebirth. Thus, you need to feel that you are in the safest, purest ceremonial space possible. Get to know who will be watching over the space and feel into who the Tata or Nana is that is holding the ceremony. Be mindful, ask questions, and listen to your inner guidance before sitting in the ceremony. Again, these can be beautiful plants to work with, but the consciousness of these plants has an intelligence of its own. Use discernment and take your time to decide whether or not you're truly open to its influence.

When we consider our other nourishing plant allies, there's no one who wouldn't benefit from partaking. They support our nervous, digestive, endocrine, respiratory, and all bodily systems. The nourishing plants like nettles, oatstraw, dandelion, linden, and many more, are a natural multivitamin when we drink them as an overnight infusion. The plants I just listed, and all herbs categorized as nourishing herbs, can be experienced daily to receive essential vitamins, and used for optimal health. I recommend that you work with one herb at a time to feel into the energy, frequency, and benefits of the plant. When you give yourself ample space, you can feel into the subtle energy of the plant and notice how you feel over time.

In the same way, instead of having one large dose of psilocybin mushrooms, where it can be difficult to integrate the experience into your practical daily life, you can microdose. You can take small doses over a period of months, and you will notice a positive impact that lasts. This trains your body and mind to seek out subtlety, which is exactly what the plants, and planet, are ever inviting us to remember. Whenever possible, seek out a professional or expert when it comes to microdosing to find out what will be right for you, your body, and your health.

When engaging with any plant, herb, medicine, mushroom, or meal, I offer a prayer to the intelligence of that which I am ingesting. I express gratitude that I get to experience it just as it gets to experience me. Instead of feeling like I am taking it, I surrender to the feeling that we coexist, in a sort of magical dance, moving into deeper alignment through, and because of, each other.

### *You Are What You Eat*

When we view our food as medicine, we will desire to have more whole foods instead of processed or fast foods. We will want to make healthy foods and slow down, chew, and digest our foods properly. Our body has receptors in our fingertips, so when we cook and eat with our hands, enzymes prepare our digestive system for intake and maximum nutrient absorption. Also, by chewing presently and mindfully, we fully break down food in our mouths. It's essential to chew long enough to kill any parasites or other unwanted guests living on our produce. However, nonorganic foods are filled with pesticides and other cancer-causing, nondigestible compounds, like wax, to make apples look shiny, something you don't want and certainly is not medicine. Modern food is what makes you need medications. Many have forgotten the simple things that give us life, losing touch of the magic that comes from knowing our connection to our First Mother and honoring her abundant, natural gifts.

We must choose healthy foods and be in right relationship with plants, herbs, and animals. When it comes to animals, some of us don't stop to imagine that the chicken on our plate was once a living creature. Sadly, modern society is completely disconnected from the process of intentional hunting. However, we do have preferences as to which animals we eat. In the Western world, we honor the life of a dog and would never think to eat Fido, but not in all places around the world. Yet we don't think twice about eating lamb, which is simply a baby sheep—and also incredibly adorable. I am not saying everyone should be vegan or vegetarian, yet I am inviting you to be conscious of your choices so that you honor the life that you are using to sustain you.

Everyone would do well with eating more plants and herbs. Indigenous cultures and your ancient Ancestors ate meat, but a key difference is they saw and respected the process of taking life. They honored the sacrifice, eating with gratitude and reverence for the life-giving bison, deer, rabbit, bear, and fish they harvested. When we feel deep gratitude, we have the opportunity to digest the nutrients more efficiently, and we will be less likely to be wasteful or gluttonous. The higher quality of foods, and especially meats, that you eat, the more you'll realize you need far less than we've been programmed to consume.

The Blood Type Diet, as popularized by Dr. Peter J. D'Adamo, proposes that people with different blood types (A, B, AB, or O) should consume different types of foods based on their ancestral diets. For some of us, being vegan or vegetarian is even more suitable for our health, especially if you have A+ or A- blood type. However, there has been a distorted agenda that has gripped Western society: the emergence of plant-based, alternative meats. Some of these contain carcinogens and are even more unhealthy than meats pumped full of hormones from cows fed genetically modified corn. Grass-fed and organic should be the only kind of meat you consume, and it's even better to eat meat from an animal you've hunted or caught. Since that's not feasible for most of our lifestyles, you can find a farm who practices humane methods of meat harvesting. These uncomfortable topics are things to know and tune in to in order to nourish your temple in the best way possible.

The plants or vegetables you eat are best fresh, unfrozen, and minimally cooked. It should feel like the food you eat was recently alive or is still raw on your plate. However, you need to make sure it is cleaned properly, and by chewing fully, you'll break your food down fully and digest efficiently. If we are truly conscious of the fact that everything is living and interconnected to us, then eating more produce full of life is optimal. Perhaps we can be less wasteful and careless about what we are consuming when we realize that our continued well-being and the fate of humanity depend on it.

This can feel like an unwinnable battle and unbearable burden when healthy foods seem to be more expensive. Eating organically is believed to be financially unobtainable for many, yet it is possible and essential. Being raised in a low-income family, I was nutrient deficient during my formative years all the way up until my early 20s. Also, I was addicted to highly processed, sugary, and oily foods. Organic foods may be more expensive in the short-term but will likely save you money from medical bills in the long-term. Even if someone doesn't have access to fresh, organic foods, being grateful for what one does have is just as impactful to how the body digests whatever it's given. Having gratitude for what plants and animals provide allows us to be conscious of and fully receive what we are taking in. Only then can we reciprocate love for what we have.

### *Consumption vs. Reciprocity*

The modern world needs a fundamental reframe of how we view, connect with, and value everything in our world. What we have been taught, especially in the Western world, is that everything should be sold for a profit, and objects with a hefty price tag or name brand hold more value. Capitalistic societies, and the people within, do not practice feeling gratitude for everything already owned. If we did, we wouldn't continue the ritual of buying more things to compensate for the programmed notions that we as individuals aren't, or don't have, enough.

There is a reason they call shopping "retail therapy." People use their purchasing power to buy more things because shopping makes them feel better for a little while. This endless cycle of reward-seeking doesn't last long and is unsustainable. Retail therapy allows someone to feel a pseudo sense of pleasure, joy, and confidence. While there's nothing wrong with treating yourself in balance and moderation, consumption won't give you what you're really looking for. All marketing tactics via advertisements, commercials, posters, billboards, etc., exist solely on the idea that you are lacking and someone or something will satisfy your need. You give away your money to someone who makes you feel like they have and can provide what you want. This is no way a dismissal of or ingratitude for the beautiful aspects of modern society; however, the subtle but critical difference is if we're engaging with it mindfully or mindlessly.

Reaching outside ourselves to feel better will never fully satisfy us. This is because marketing and capitalism operate on dopamine being the hormone we've become addicted to. Dopamine is the "reward chemical," and you get it from completing a task, eating food, or celebrating something. So, going out on a "quest" and buying clothes, eating food, and celebrating yourself with a new item are dopamine-seeking activities. Dopamine-fueled joy doesn't last, whereas oxytocin, serotonin, and endorphin are much more sustainable hormones. Remember, drinking ceremonial cacao supports you in feeling sustainable bliss and joy—a much better choice than a high-sugar, carcinogenic Caramel Macchiato from Starbucks.

We have learned to mask our authentic longings by indulging in consumerism, which offers a quick hit of dopamine. This makes us feel more alive and fulfilled, but only for a fleeting moment. We can't skip over our feelings, our true likes, or our dislikes. That's why we have to know ourselves to experience true bliss. You have to feel it to heal it. Whenever you feel the need for a dopamine hit, dig deeper and you'll probably find a sense of lack from not feeling comfortable, loved, safe, or cared for. This is the perfect opportunity to seek out serotonin, also called the "mood stabilizer." You can build serotonin within yourself from sunlight, going on a walk, meditating, drinking cacao, or eating dark chocolate! After meditating and drinking cacao, you can exercise or use essential oils to release endorphins, your natural "pain killer." Finally, playing with a dog, giving someone a hug, holding hands, or being intimate releases oxytocin, the "love hormone."

Whether it's cacao, essential oils, sunlight, a puppy, or a beloved, life is here to support your healing. Plants and animals are here as allies to help you feel deeply grateful for who you are and what you have. And this gratitude can inspire you to give back to everything around you. This is the principle of reciprocity in action—something that was inherent to our Indigenous Ancestors.

We can give back in big and small ways. If you have a womb and are bleeding, you can bleed on the Earth to give nutrients to the soil. We can compost our leftover foods to create fertilizer for the soil. We can farm regeneratively so that we do not destroy the planet but use sustainable practices to steward the land and grow our foods. Money and plants are both forms of energy. How you use them can uplift others, bring your health into alignment, and heal the planet. Consider donating to local regenerative farmers, invest in a traditional herbalism course, and find other creative ways to use your purchasing power for your own and the greater good.

The ancient Maya, as well as modern shamans and midwives, Tatas and Nanas, live in a natural state of gratitude for all things. Gratitude, reciprocity, and reverence are at the forefront of how Indigenous peoples live in right relation with all that is. Sacred incense like copal, a tree resin, has been used for thousands of years to purify the air, connect with the unseen realms, and is burned as an offering. As I shared previously, cacao has also been a staple of Mayan culture, even being used as a form of currency. Cacao is literally liquid gold! One of the most popular remaining codices, the Popol Vuh, describes how in the Mayan creation myth, humans were created from maize (corn). It's clear to see how central plants were to the ancient Maya and still continue to be for Native peoples. We are wise to learn from these simple, easy, and essential ways. By embracing these traditions and respecting the deep connection between humans and the natural world, we can enrich our own lives while also honoring the wisdom that has been passed down through generations.

There is a simple but incredible wisdom available to us when we live in harmony with plants, animals, and all the planet's gifts. Not only are plants highly practical and essential for our well-being, but they are magical, indefinable, and their intelligence requires us to get out of our heads and into our hearts. They serve as worlds within themselves that we are privileged to get to experience. They soothe us, energize us, and remind us of that which we cannot see with just our two eyes, offering a divine, and often delicious, reminder of how good it truly is to be human.

### *Embodiment Practice: Cacao Ceremony*

My favorite way to connect with a plant's intelligence is by creating a cacao ceremony. A cacao ceremony is a very gentle yet profound heart-opening experience. In a ceremony, I begin by burning sustainably harvested herbs or incense. Look up what herbs your Ancestors used or those that grow locally. Common sacred herbs are sage, lavender, cedar, rosemary, sweetgrass, and many others. Burn the herbs and call in your loving Ancestors, guides, angels, and protectors to be with you.

I then prepare the cacao, playing medicine or meditative music. For a ceremonial dose, I use about one ounce of Somalux ceremonial cacao that is already chopped, or I chop up the block myself. I add hot water; spices like cinnamon, nutmeg, and ginger; coconut milk, sometimes coconut butter for more creaminess, and natural sweetener like monk fruit or coconut sugar. I either place all these into a blender or in a pot on the stove. It's about as simple as making a cup of hot chocolate, yet this will feel far different if you sit with your cup with presence and intention. I usually drink cacao in the morning, as a rising ritual to support my meditations and creativity, yet I've shared it in a group ceremony with as few as one other person up to hundreds at once. I suggest meditating, praying, or dancing to tap into the available magic and guidance from both seen and unseen positive forces. Doing this outdoors makes the experience even more meaningful, as you're sharing it with the natural elements like trees, plants, and rocks.

If you feel emotional, you may want to cry; if you feel silly, you may laugh and want to giggle, or you may sweat, dance, or sing. You may want to go within by meditating or journaling. You might not feel anything at all the first time. Whatever you feel is perfect. Give yourself space to allow whatever needs to come through. Simply let yourself feel deeply into what is present for you. Remember that the magic is in the mundane, so train yourself to value subtlety. Remember to give thanks to your spirit guides, spirit animals, the loving Ancestors, Mother Nature, and the Creator. When you feel complete with the ceremony, take a few deep cleansing breaths, ground into the soil beneath you, and feel how deeply your roots are reaching. From there, go about your day from a centered and relaxed place.

### *It's Tea Time, Innit?*

Another way to connect with plants is to make herbal tea, prepare an overnight infusion of nourishing herbs, or take a bath with herbs. Try each of these practices on different days. When you are ready to work with cacao, I recommend my cacao, Somalux, because it is prepared intentionally and by Indigenous women's collectives that I've been supporting in Guatemala for many years. If you are making tea, use organic, local, or sustainable herbs. Like a cacao ceremony, choose to sit with a nourishing plant that calls to you. Give yourself space to feel whatever wants to come through. Sit and meditate with the tea while listening to relaxing music or soaking in the silence. Again, let yourself feel deeply with the assistance of the plant. Invite the plant to experience you as you experience it, and welcome whatever wisdom or guidance the plant has for you.

If you are making an herbal bath, first you want to steep the tea for 10 to 15 minutes and then, with a strainer or through a French press, pour the tea into the bath without the herbs. Using a couple drops of essential oils is another great way to be supported by plants. However, make sure you are using oils that are okay to use topically on your skin, like lavender, rose, eucalyptus, or lemongrass. After your bath, give the wet herbs to the soil as an offering and to the land you live on.

CHAPTER 7:

# Return to the Mother

*"Then our grandmother said, 'Here I am; I am the one who gives life.' Soon after that, there emerged from the water a multitude of men and women who were able to talk, look, listen, walk, and grasp things. They were made of yellow and white maize dough [ . . . ]."*

— Popol Vuh

*"And Jehovah God formed man of the dust of the ground and breathed into his nostrils the breath of life; and man became a living soul."*

— Genesis 2:7, the Bible

Many of us have been conditioned to view ourselves as separate from nature, rather than as an integral part of it. With over 56 percent of the global population living in cities, we see the natural world as out there, foreign, or something we just visit briefly. Nature is often something we tolerate, and it can seem to inconvenience us more often than it supports us. Rain could ruin plans, high winds could take down power lines, and if you drop your phone into water, you're left without navigation, music, and many other extraordinary conveniences.

Yet staying connected to the natural world promotes our well-being. It's our disconnection from Mother Earth that perpetuates cycles of suffering and prevents us from realizing the fullness of who we truly are. But while this disconnection seems real, the deepest truth is that it's simply a perception of being separate. Since humans have a greater ability to manipulate the environment around us, it's easier to forget we are a part of it. Humans have complex languages, culture, and a drive to rapidly expand upon or build new things. We've created culture, art, and architecture as models of what is around us. But over time, we have forgotten that what we've created is just a reflection of the things we see around us in Nature. As humans, our ability to manifest complex things makes us a unique species. This can be our greatest superpower or cause us the greatest suffering.

We forget that all things not only come from Nature, but we are Nature. We are not just from Earth, we are Earth. Our body and blood are formed from the very soils we walk upon. Being alive subjects us to challenges and dangers, yet adopting a perspective rooted in hopefulness and gratitude can transform our perception of the world from a scary place to one that is fundamentally safe. This doesn't mean bad things can't or won't happen, but witnessing the world through a lens of hopefulness and gratitude allows us to highlight and see more of the beauty amid the inherent struggles. When we grow and thrive despite our traumas, we claim our birthright as grateful beings living on a thriving planet.

As a note: You will notice in this book that we use words like Gaia, the planet, Mother Nature, or the soil instead of saying Earth as often as we can. Words hold power in their meaning, and the etymology of *Earth* means "to plow, uproot, and extract." This carries an energy of taking and destroying instead of tending to, honoring, or cultivating. We want to use words intentionally that are harmonious, so *Earth* is an example of a word that is used often but is not fully understood for what energy it carries.

## *Honoring the Journey, Living in Gratitude*

As a human being, you stand as the perfect reflection of the macrocosmic universe and microscopic organisms. There are more atoms in your body than stars in the known universe. This means there are living worlds within worlds on every level, from the minute to the magnificent. Humans have developed telescopes to see farther and microscopes to look closer, captivated with discovering every layer of life. There is an ancient principle that encapsulates this phenomenon that states, "As above, so below. As within, so without." Your human body is the Universe's mirror that it uses to know itself. We are intrinsically interconnected to all things, from distant galaxies and the billions of stars within them, to the trillions of atoms that have formed your physical body. From the soil to the stars and everything in between, you are connected to it all because you are a part of it all. When this is deeply understood, you become aware of your impact on others and are motivated to live in a manner that honors the significance of life.

It is essential to foster a healthy relationship with our inner and outer worlds to live in harmony with all things. Indigenous teachings have taught us to walk in gratitude, reverence, and reciprocity. Giving thanks keeps our body healthy and connected to the fact that being alive is a gift. Giving thanks to the things outside of us is reciprocity for the gifts that sustain our lives. The water, rocks, plants, and animals can feel our gratitude, and we too are affected by our own state of gratitude. When we live in gratitude, show thanks, and give back, we can live in right relation for all that we are provided for.

Everything is interconnected by the delicate threads of the web of life, previously understood as magic and now known as the emergent science of quantum mechanics. To live in harmony, we must be balanced within ourselves, since we are the reflection of the worlds above, below, within, and around us. To stay balanced means we must give in return for all that we receive. Mother Nature and the Universe are always conspiring in our favor and giving to us in ways seen and unseen. When we honor Nature and the gift of life; we are not parasitic to the ecosystem. Taking, draining, and only ever wanting more, we rarely stop to think of how much of a burden we have become to our Mother that just keeps giving. However, much like when a baby jaguar becomes too greedy at the teat, a Mother Jaguar will eventually swat the baby away. So many of us have only learned how to pillage and take from Nature, not even knowing that's what we're doing. We go to jobs, extracting as much money as we can from them, and our supervisors extract as much production via our time, energy, and life-force as they can.

Modern society has not learned how to commune and live in reverence to all worlds. The living world is patiently waiting for us to awaken to Her power and therefore, our own potential. She gifts us plants to remind us of our connection. She sings songs to us through the wind. Her heartbeat is a drum that gives us passion and rhythm. Her rivers invite us to purify, her mountains enrapture us, and her fires inspire us, yet most still do not appreciate Her. It takes practice to remember. We humans so easily forget, and that is why it is essential to practice gratitude, making every moment a ceremony for our continued remembering.

Being disconnected from Nature disempowers us and places our power into the hands of an authority that governs how we should live our lives. When we come back into connection with our body, mind, soul, and the natural world around us, we regain our inherent power. Our ability to create society as a model of life has led us to forget the simple, healthy ways of being that our ancient Ancestors knew. Remembering does not mean we try to go back and be as they were, but we learn from those who made mistakes, as well as those who were successful. We all must do our best, allowing us to move forward in a beautiful way by honoring the journey and living in gratitude.

### *Divine Intelligence*

Everything in Nature happens in cycles. For plants, animals, and humans, the cycle of the seasons affect us physically, but also emotionally. When spring arrives, we are more energized alongside everything bursting with life. In this season, we can clean out the old, create new projects, and blossom. In the summer, the sun is at its peak, we have more energy, and are more apt to travel but can often feel overwhelmed from the heat. Summertime is a party, a time to celebrate with intention and balance. Autumn comes and things begin to slow down as we prepare for the cold. This is a season to harvest the fruits of your hard work and enjoy the sweetness of life. Autumn reminds us that letting go can be a beautiful process, like the green leaves transforming into vibrant rainbows of light. Once winter sets in, it brings more darkness and slowness. This is a restful, introspective period. We are wise to learn from the animals and go deep within ourselves, having an energetic hibernation until spring.

Even in a single day, all four seasons happen. Immediately upon waking, you are in spring, the most creative part of your day. If you rested well and took care of yourself the previous day, you'll wake feeling refreshed with a natural high. Before looking at your phone, doing any work, or accomplishing any task, the early morning is where new ideas can arise. If you don't experience this, then you're likely bringing in residue from past actions that are making your morning foggy, groggy, and unpleasant. As spring turns to summer, you begin to heat up and have more energy. This is where you can eat, work, and get on with your day-to-day tasks. When the sun is high, remember to not burn yourself out. As your day begins to shift into autumn, allow yourself to transition into more stillness. It can be tempting to power through this season of the day with caffeine or other stimulants. But if you do so, you'll miss out on the sweetness of good, deep, and nourishing sleep later at night. As darkness of twilight sets in, make yourself cozy, warm, and safe. Review your day. Reflect on what you're grateful for and what you can do to build upon the positive momentum of that day. And then go to sleep, without any technology well before bedtime, hibernating in full gratitude that tomorrow you will get to wake and continue living life.

Rest is an essential phase that supports our growth and healing. When we rest, we integrate the knowledge we've gained into our body. In meditations, daydreams, or short naps, insights or inspiration comes to us. This is a complete reframe from Western culture where people find their value and worth through pushing through tiredness, always doing more, and focusing only on accomplishing. This way of creating comes from a deep sense of lack, and regardless of what we do, what we have, or what we feel, it will not be enough.

If we listen when our body asks for rest and give it the medicine it needs, we'll experience a sense of renewal. Even after bouts of illness, I feel as if I've been through an initiation where I come out the other side reborn. Once, after getting intense food poisoning in Bali, I made it a priority to rest and recover. Instead of trying to power through, I went to the hospital to get IV fluids and gave myself time to simply be with the sickness. In the week that followed, I started receiving downloads, ideas, and core themes for this book. I was able to receive guidance from the unseen dimensions and from Spirit that would have been undiscovered had I tried to rush the process of rest and recovery. I didn't work on the book during that time, but afterward, I had more clarity and inspiration than before.

Our ancient Ancestors knew and prioritized the importance of rest. In the Mayan Haab' Calendar, which is their 365-day calendar, they have five days called Wayeb. These five closing days of the year are considered "days out of time," which are a time of rest before the beginning of the next year. Wayeb happens in February of the Gregorian calendar, as the Northern Hemisphere comes into springtime, which is naturally the true New Year. Wayeb is considered an important time to take time off work, lighten up on exercising, and be with oneself in a deep way. Doing so, you wrap up the year and go into the next one with fresh eyes and an open heart. It gives us time to recognize what we've done, what we're going to do better, and feel into what worked and what didn't. This is a time for compassion, ease, rest, reflection, forgiveness, and prayer—a season to give thanks for all things. Wayeb is considered a day without government, so it's our responsibility to guide ourselves during this time and be mindful of how we spend our energy and time. This supports us in staying balanced, gentle, and focused on our own energy.

Rest is especially important for women during their period. When hormones are properly balanced through lifestyle, diet, and environment, it's natural to bleed in sync with full or new moons. As we move through our cycles, it is wise to listen to what our body is communicating. Not only does bleeding follow the phases of the moon, the four yearly seasons also happen during each menstrual period. When we are in our luteal phase, or coming into our moon phase, it is like autumn where we should slow down and flow more gently. When we are heavily bleeding, we are in our winter phase and should rest, nourish our bodies, tend to our inner world, and be gentle with ourselves. During this season, giving your blood back to the soil is an incredibly empowering practice because you are sharing your sacred life-force back in reciprocity to the Earth. You are feeding the soil with blood that's high in stem cells and healing plasma. You are simultaneously reprogramming yourself with the understanding that your blood is beautiful, healing, and powerful. When we are in our follicular phase, it is our spring phase, and we should become more active and move that building energy. In our ovulation phase, this is our summer and a time for us to harness powerful life-force energy that is most potent at that time. Use this energy to birth and create things into being.

### *Feminine Intelligence*

All human life begins as a biological female embryo in the womb, and through the introduction of the Y chromosome, it transitions into a biological male. Therefore, there is a fundamental feeling of separation that defines life as a man, whether they're aware of it or not. The key is for boys and men to be given the tools, environment, and support to recognize how these feelings of separation manifest. Since all men come from a woman, as an embryo and also from their mother, there is a core "shadow" that every man must bring into the light or be unconsciously controlled by it. This is the feeling of "not being enough."

Women often struggle with the pervasive belief that they are "too much," a message frequently reinforced by societies shaped by imbalanced men. However, for us to recognize our own body is a conduit between different realms, with the portal between worlds between our thighs, no external opinion can detract from our inherent worth or diminish the fact that we are a divine expression of the Creator. We can give birth to life and sustain it, a power no man will ever know. Women are the embodiment of Mother Nature and the physical manifestation of divine magic. Women are beautiful, soft, delicate, wild, tough, and strong. Like the planet, we are made of earth, air, water, and fire, soft and resilient, delicate yet strong, and we sustain and nourish the world with our bounties. A woman is a woman, and no number of physical alterations makes someone more of a woman or less of a woman.

What would happen if all women were praised for our magical ways? What would the world look like if Mother Nature was honored for her likeness to a woman's inherent beauty? I have wondered what our society would look like if we had a matriarchy. I believe that's what we need to restore balance. Since we are so far off balance, in order to right the wrongs and reorient ourselves, we need a systemic adoption of matriarchy, supported by healthy forms of patriarchy, to course correct. What we ultimately want is an egalitarian society, but we will need to see a fundamental shift in honor and reverence of the feminine, the Mother, the planet, and all beings before we can truly call our world a safe place for all.

This shift could begin by making Earth Day on April 22 a nationally recognized holiday, where everyone is given a day off work. Instead of buying fireworks and exploding masculine gunpowder in the skies and littering all over the soils, we create things to gift our First Mother with. We could give a song, a dance, a poem, a bouquet of wildflowers, a dessert, a cake, or hot cacao, giving back to Her in reverence. Can you imagine what an entire nation in reverence to the Mother would look and feel like? I think it's time we make major holidays in honor and celebration of the waters, rocks, stars, the moon, our Ancestors, sunrises, the elements, directions, birth, death, and so much more. There is so much our planet gives us to honor and celebrate!

When we are disconnected from our First Mother, we live out of balance and without integrity. We've forgotten how to live in harmony, and instead perpetrate disrespect and dishonor to the feminine and to the Mother that sustains us. As we're indoctrinated into family patterning and current patriarchal societies, we forget that a relationship between Mother and child is one filled with love and defined by reciprocity. Mother gives her milk, and the baby energetically gives unconditional love in return, with oxytocin flowing abundantly between them.

The only way to make real change and make the world a better place is to transform ourselves. We first do this by honoring, loving, and caring for the feminine aspects within us. Feminine beings deserve to know that they are the embodiment of Mother Earth's beauty and power, thus treating themselves, their sisters, and their brothers with unconditional love. Masculine beings get to learn how to honor, cherish, revere, and uplift the feminine that has been suppressed. For too long, masculine hierarchies have pushed down and shamed the feminine for our inherent beauty, sensuality, and power. There is no surprise that there is a clear reflection between the way we treat both women and the planet.

We shed harmful programming when we heal from within and begin to live authentically. This is an ongoing process that includes self-awareness, education, and action, yet we get to relax and know that we do not have to do anything perfectly. Simply showing up authentically is a gift and balm for the wounds of this world. The only frequency that is a higher vibration than gratitude is authenticity. This means being true to yourself, regardless of the specific feeling you're feeling. It could be anger, sadness, grief, or gratitude—whatever you feel, by feeling it fully, you'll be in tune with the Universe and honoring what it truly means to be human.

Since our society is disconnected from ourselves, each other, the land, and the elements, it's no surprise that so many people are unappreciative of life. We are out of sync with the true essence of life. It's our sacred responsibility to remember our connection to all things so we can live in reciprocity. Reciprocity—the fundamental essence of feminine intelligence—is what takes place when we give offerings at all things. It is the exchange of things for mutual benefit. Our Ancestors knew the power of gratitude and practiced reciprocity with all things, leading them to live harmoniously.

The foundation of what we now know as economy was not bartering, trading, or capitalism. It was one of trust, community, and reciprocity. It was a system of, "I've got your back, and next time you got mine." If a fisherman caught excess, he would share his fish with others without payment. The next time someone, let's say a weaver, had an extra shirt, they'd reciprocate their goods back to the fisherman. This type of economy requires trust between people. In modern times, money acts as the exchange of trust. If you have an object of value, I can give you money, which reciprocates value back to you. However, exchange with money, and subsequently markets, industry, and capitalism, opens itself to manipulation, greed, and hoarding. The ancient Maya used cacao as a form of currency. Cacao was literally liquid gold. But using a natural object as a standardized form of value meant that there is no benefit to hoarding it. Someone could keep as much as they could for themself, but after a couple years, they would be left with nothing after the cacao spoiled.

The beauty of reciprocity is that when we give, we receive so much in return. Being in the state of giving for the sake of giving, we connect to a bigger force than just ourselves. The magic of gratitude is that when we give thanks, in turn, we are given more to be grateful for. When we live in this way, we are trusting, open, and supporting those around us. If we all lived in an authentically grateful and reciprocal way, the structures and systems that exist would crumble. When we heal ourselves, the worlds within and around us heal as well.

### *Sensuality Is Natural*

A woman's body is a beautiful reflection of the planet's full-spectrum aliveness. She is dynamic, voluptuous, curvy, juicy, and bursting with all expressions of life. Witnessing an empowered woman in her sensuality is as natural as revering Mother Earth's inherent beauty. It's also an opportunity to work through conditioning around women using their voice, showing their skin, and not being free to be big and take up space.

If we feel ourselves judging a woman's sensuality, what does that bring up? What does her free expression elicit within? What if her pleasure and empowerment elicit a feeling of inspiration instead of separation? Can we remember that sensual expression is natural and is simply life-force energy flowing through? Can we reprogram our minds to see sensuality as something natural and life-giving? When we judge another, it's simply revealing to us a place within us that hasn't been acknowledged. Understanding this, our judgments are an opportunity to check in with ourselves and see with eyes of the heart.

Empowering the expression of sacred sensuality is critical because it instantly dissolves misogyny, patriarchy, and inequality. However, it's important to clarify that I'm not talking about a hypersexualized, leaky type of lust-seeking energy that needs external validation. That's another type of energy. I'm talking about that liberated, loving, and unashamed owning of your body, blissed out by the way your hips sway to a good song, and using your velvety voice when sweet, juicy fruit touches your lips. Sacred sensuality is beautiful when coming from a pure and empowered place. It's not seeking to get anything from anyone, but rather being in the most vulnerable expression of one's truth. There is also a difference between pornographic content and the pure expression of innate beauty. The difference is felt and recognizable to someone living from the heart.

It's also important to highlight that sensuality is a way of living. Sensuality is the enjoyment, expression, or pursuit of physical pleasures. It is to be fully alive and in touch with your senses. When you see a beautiful flower, taste a ripe fruit, or take in a sunset, you're engaging with the cosmic eroticism that fills every moment. True enlightenment is not being emotionless toward the pleasures of life, but an uninhibited expression of gratitude for the minute and magnificent, the subtle and the serene. Expressing gratitude amid feeling pleasure for the fullness of what life provides us is what the human experience is all about. This is why, for the Maya, gratitude was the key that unlocked the mysteries of life.

### *Conclusion*

The Sacred Mayan Calendar brings valuable wisdom when it comes to understanding our life path. It encapsulates all energies on Earth through the 20 Nawals and the 13 numbers, showing us the different varieties that co-create reality. The Nawals carry different energies like leaders, artists, healers, prayer makers, or law keepers. In Western society, what comes naturally to us gets swept aside in favor of finding a career that brings the most success or financial gain. In order for us to live in harmony and live in a balanced community, we've got to know ourselves better and work with what comes naturally to us. When we honor our natural talents, we will live in harmony within ourselves and bring value to our community. This is how we can be good at something and find success with what we love doing. Knowing this can guide us on our life path, in relationships, when we've reached a crossroads, or when we don't know what to do next in our professional lives. It can also be helpful to determine what may come easy for children so that we may guide them in a way that brings out their gifts.

With your Mayan chart, you have nine different Nawals that influence you. My Mayan Sign is 3 Ajpu, which represents the sun, the path to the Divine, and the mystical realms. It is the most shamanic of the Nawals, yet it is not the most desirable for even the eldest of spiritual guides. That is because one must undergo many challenges to emerge from the darkness in order to shine like the sun. In the beginning of 2022, I lost my grandma and a baby within weeks of each other. I endured a tremendous amount of stress, sadness, and grief. I stumbled and made mistakes, but I continued to get up and do my best to do and be better. It was the hardest year of my life, yet it grew me, taught me, and expanded my capacity for more love. We cannot access new heights, new levels of love, without also feeling the depths of grief and pain that also exist. That year I had the most breakthroughs and realizations, and this book was birthed in the midst of it all.

For me, the energy of Ajpu shifts into Q'anil as I begin to embody my eldership. Although I will always be Ajpu and predominantly have that energy, I will become more influenced by Q'anil. This is a very fortunate Nawal, one that is abundant and prosperous. While my journey has been incredibly challenging, my path has been paved with so much beauty, bliss, and pleasure. We all have aspects that are supportive to help us clear our unique karma, develop our persona, and live our specific dharma. To overcome our challenges and begin to thrive, we must turn to the intelligence of nature. Thankfully, the Maya encoded the wisdom of nature into their Sacred Calendar, and now we have the privilege of turning to this wisdom to support us. To make this accessible for many more, in 2025, we will publish a Mayan Oracle Deck that also can be used as a daily Mayan Calendar to support you in learning about each Nawal and each number's unique energy.

Indigenous teachings show us that each person has a unique gift to contribute to the whole community. Some may have a proclivity for health and wellness, creativity, singing, hunting, gathering, protecting, healing, leading, planning, or negotiating. This creates balance within our communities. Like I shared in the previous chapters, the Mayan Sacred Calendar supports us in knowing our personalities, our weaknesses, and our strengths. The calendar provides us with the combination of the number and the Nawal, which determines your personality, your strengths, and your weaknesses. It outlines your past, present, and future, as well as your feminine and masculine energies—it's a holistic approach to self-discovery.

In contrast to Nature-based traditions, Western religions say you must do something to be saved. The divine intelligence of Nature reminds you that you are innately sacred. Religion is often used to your power, while living in harmony with nature keeps you empowered. Religion encourages separation, yet Nature reminds you that we are one with all. Yes, Spirit moves through all channels, so I know there are some beautiful examples of loving, religious-based communities. Yet you don't have to go into a building or have another person be your intermediary to access God; your backyard, a tree, a river, or a rock are all divine temples that we are wise to return to.

### *Embodiment Practice: Grounding in Nature*

Someone once asked a Lakota medicine woman for the cure to heal from disease, stress, and trauma. She replied with the simplest of answers: "Go out into Nature." She went on to share that being immersed in an intimate way with Nature healed her anxiety, loneliness, and depression.

Many studies show that grounding, meaning placing your bare feet or hands on the ground, for at least an hour every day significantly boosts your health. When you walk on the ground barefoot and your feet directly touch the soils, your skin absorbs negative electrons, which helps to balance your body's positive electrons. This exchange balances your internal bioelectrical environment, relaxes you, and stabilizes your circadian rhythm. You will see improvements in your health when you practice grounding daily. The more we practice, the more we will remember that we are interconnected with Nature.

However, it's important to realize that when we receive from Nature, we can benefit from giving an offering. This is a beautiful example of living in right relation and reciprocity. Offer something natural, biodegradable, and something that you value. It can be as little as a flower, or you can make a meal, tea, or leave incense burning outside. When we give offerings, we are placing ourselves in humility and reverence for what we are given. Each day we wake, we're given so much to be grateful for. If you really tried to count your blessings, you'd do so for infinity.

Each day, go into Nature. Feel your toes touch the grass, dirt, sand, or mud. Give yourself time to rest here. Meditate on the ground. Allow yourself to get wet, sandy, or dirty. Feel yourself supported by our Great Mother. Go for a walk in nature and take notice of all the elements that surround you. Dance with the elements of wind and earth. Feel the sun on your skin absorbing vitamin D, which is vital for your health as well. How do you feel when you walk among the trees? Can you take the biggest breath you've taken all day, and allow your exhale to be an offering of gratitude to the trees around you?

Give thanks and be outside with nature daily. Rest in the Great Mothers embrace; you will heal while you rest and remember yourself here.

CHAPTER 8:

# Rising from the Ashes

*"You may encounter many defeats,*
*but you must not be defeated. In fact,*
*it may be necessary to encounter the defeats,*
*so you can know who you are, what you can*
*rise from, how you can still come out of it."*

— Maya Angelou

Fire is magical and transformational, a light amid what would be utter darkness. Fire is the pure energy of the Divine, for in the beginning, all life begins as a spark. The exact moment you were conceived, and your father's sperm met your mother's egg in the womb, sparks flew. An explosion of zinc occurs when a human egg is activated by sperm enzymes. The intensity of the sparks indicates the egg's potential to develop into a healthy embryo, meaning the brighter the light, the greater presence of potential life! Fire is the primordial energy that gives life to matter. From the moment you're born till the moment you transition into death, your heart pulses with electricity, your neurons fire, and your breath gives fuel to your inner flame.

Fire is the very first element, and the rest of the physical world is born from its pure essence. All elements of matter like hydrogen, nitrogen, and all others on the periodic table are forged under tremendous pressure and heat in the furnaces of stars. All things have been created because of fire, and in turn, fire can destroy all things. Fire is the only thing that could destroy everything on the entire planet. If a large enough ball of fire impacted the Earth, via an asteroid or a nuclear explosion, all living things could be wiped out and are unlikely to recover for a very long time. Water has, and could again, cover the entire surface of the planet, but things would be simply submerged. Fire entirely transforms.

Fire is the purest element of them all because it cannot be touched by the human hand. The planet, the winds, and the waters have experienced deep distress, disrespect, and pollution, almost to the point of irreversible destruction. Unlike these elements that have been contaminated by humans in all types of ways, fire cannot be tainted or polluted by anything. While the smoke from fire can contain pollutants from burning chemicals or waste, fire itself is eternally, unchangeably pure.

Fire is a mysterious paradox, for it holds the full spectrum of light, yet it casts shadows. Fire is purity and it is destruction. It is light, but whatever it burns turns to darkened ash. What can we make of this mystery that light and dark go hand-in-hand, that burning stars in the sky can only be seen because of the ocean of darkness that surrounds them? How do we interact with something holding such ancient power? With utter reverence and religious awe. However, if instead of reverence we are filled with fear, we can be consumed by fire. What we want is a perfect balance; to be filled with passion, but not too much that we get burned.

Fire teaches us that we, too, hold purity and destruction, the light and the dark, both victim and perpetrator, fuel and flame. We hold the whole spectrum within us and cast shadows as a result; this is what it means to be alive. The fire reminds us that it is our sacred responsibility to purify our thoughts and actions so we do not become destructive or get lost in the darkness. If you listen to what life has to teach you through the simplicity of the elements, you'll find you're just as powerful as they are, because they've made you and you are them. Being a spark amid the darkness is the most ancient remembrance of yourself, for it's through the purity of the fire in your mother's womb that your soul entered into this realm.

### *Tend to Your Fire Tenderly*

Fire within our body gives life to our beating heart. On the other end of the spectrum, if our internal fire rages within us, we'll be consumed with anger. If we use fire to empower us, it is life-giving. If we ignore it or let it build up within, it will burn us to the ground. Anger is like any other emotion. It isn't good or bad; it simply exists. We must acknowledge its existence so that it does not have any power over us. The more we avoid our anger, the bigger our inner fire will rage. The bigger the flame, the bigger the shadow. So, if we don't regulate ourselves, each triggering or angering experience will only add more fuel to the fire. When we stop denying or avoiding our angry emotions, we can let our anger have its natural expression in a way that is not projecting onto or destructive to others, but rather allow it to transform and renew us.

Anger is an emotion that is culturally frowned upon. People don't know what to do with the "angry woman." Sweet and kind women who do not get angry or emotional have been praised in our society. As such, we have been programmed for millennia to sit down and shut up instead of letting our anger fuel us and speak up for ourselves. I know firsthand how common it is to feel judged and shamed for feeling or showing anger. It is far more accepting for men to get angry, proven by the saying "boys will be boys," but for women, it is unladylike to express too much emotion. It's normalized for men to be explosive, direct, and determined, but when a woman is, she's considered bitchy or "too much."

It's important to note that boys who grow up without being supported in feeling their emotions, shown by the phrase "men don't cry," harden their hearts. We all naturally feel sadness and anger, but if we show it, we're often seen as too sensitive or dramatic. All of this is blatantly incorrect. Humans have a lot to be angry about! Children have a lot to be sad about. Adults have a lot to be stressed about. Suppressing our anger, people pleasing, or fawning is a conditioned coping mechanism that we must stop perpetuating if we want to experience the fullness of life. All people have the right to feel all of their feelings, and express them in constructive ways, even if at first it seems messy, "too much," or uncomfortable to witness.

For many years, I wasn't ready to feel my deeper emotions because I didn't have the capacity or emotional safety to sit with anything too heavy. Instead of feeling my anger, I would use things to distract myself and push down my feelings. I did my best with the tools I had, but there came a time when I realized bypassing my anger and other difficult emotions wasn't helping me. Instead of feeling it all, I'd throw a blanket over everything with motivational, positive, or affirming thoughts. Bypassing anger doesn't make it disappear. It's like putting a Band-Aid on a gaping wound within the heart. We have to feel our feelings. It may feel scary and messy at first, but in the long-term, it's well worth it. And now that you've read the earlier chapters, you have the tools to feel regulated and safe while feeling any feelings that come.

This anger that I felt to my core was so strong at times that it felt bigger than just my own, more than from what I'd experienced in this lifetime to be sure. Children are born with over 400 preconditioned traits, reaching far back into their entire lineage. Parents make the most impact, but each one of us is a mosaic of all those who came before us. We know that we are given an inheritance of both helpful and unhelpful traits passed down through our lineage. Unresolved karmic patterns of anger, resentment, addiction, or abuse are embedded into our DNA.

Imagine what the Ancestors experienced after surviving colonization. They had no choice but to assimilate to survive. There is no doubt that many were seething with both anger and grief. To survive, they would have had to ignore their feelings and push it down just like many of us still do today. Millions, and maybe even billions, of people have not been able to fully process or find resolution for troublesome feelings. Yet it is more natural to feel, grieve, and let go of what we cannot control.

I come from a heritage of both the wise and the wounded. We all do. We have Ancestors within our lineage who were powerful healers, artists, weavers, and warriors. And because of harmful forms of patriarchy, collectively we've had mothers and grandmothers who were wounded, bullied, and taken from, forcing them to suppress their anger that was powerful enough to burn everything to the ground. Many women were, and metaphorically still are, burned at the stake, used as examples of the dangers of being too much.

My maternal grandmother stayed busy, always cleaning, always doing, never too relaxed; unable to slow down, receive loving touch, or feel safe enough to simply be. She had much anger within her for reasons known and unknown. Her behavior was that of a deeply traumatized person, passed down through the mothers and grandmothers before her, and intensified by her own difficult life. She didn't show this side to all people, for she was beloved by her immediate and extended family. But those closest to her could feel her sadness and anger.

I remember when she would be angry with my grandfather, cursing him in Spanish and leaving a palpable negativity in the air. The anger she carried was dense, heavy, and she couldn't forgive or let it go. Yet like us all, she carried the full spectrum within her. She had so much beauty in her; she was loved and admired by thousands. She had a generous heart with everyone that she came across, always taking care of others but never truly giving love to herself or fully accepting love from others. Every time I wanted to give her a long hug, she'd tap my back with an indication that it was long enough and too intimate for her comfort.

Sadly, she passed away from Alzheimer's, which came out of nowhere but took her life within a year. Her anger hardened her heart and mind, causing the illness that led to her untimely death, shocking everyone that she passed before my grandfather. She used to be as healthy as an ox, strong, and hardworking, but she died from her inability to feel safe, find stillness, or release her inner fire in constructive ways. This is why I choose to feel the fire, explore my shadows, and heal my heart so that I stay tender and open. I heal for myself, my grandmothers before me, and a legacy of love that I choose to continue.

It is our divine responsibility to acknowledge our difficult feelings and heal our hearts, for ourselves, the Ancestors who could not do this work before us, and for generations to come. We shine light on our shadows so that fear, anger, jealousy, greed, and other destructive emotions lose their power over us. First, we acknowledge that our pain exists without trying to figure out where those feelings come from. We then allow ourselves to feel our feelings without trying to change them or project them onto anything or anyone outside of us. We accept that anger, like all emotions, exists, and we integrate that "shadow" with loving kindness.

Through this process you must hold yourself and others with care and gentleness. Feel it all, but do not steep in anger for too long or you will feel burned. If you simply let the anger exist, it will transform not only what you're upset with but your own identification with what troubles you. You can do this as slowly as you need; you do not need to go fast. When you feel feelings of anger come up, remember to breathe, be with it, and then express it. Go for a brisk walk, shake, run, work out, or rage out. A rage ritual is shared at the end of this chapter for you to practice this in a conscious and healing way.

Your anger can be life-giving or destructive. If you direct the fires of transformation toward helping you heal, you can burn away old stories that aren't serving the highest purpose for your life. Oftentimes, when we finally let ourselves feel our anger, we find that underneath there is a well of sadness that has been waiting to be uncovered.

Anger gives way to sadness and grief. Sadness and grief, when felt fully, leads to finding an opportunity to give yourself or someone else love. Trace back every emotion, every action, every reaction, and you will find love or a seeking to be loved at the core of all of life.

In this process, sometimes heavier emotions can feel like they're too much to deal with, but remember to turn to the tools you have learned in this book. Come to your breath, your heart, the plants, Great Spirit, and your unconditionally loving Ancestors. You are never alone and always supported, whether you can see it or not.

### *Full-Spectrum Aliveness*

Those who shine the brightest have been forged in the fire. I know some incredible women and men who are truly pure and radiant beings, yet they did not get there because they were always that way, nor was it easy. Things weren't always perfect, nor have they always been shining. Their lives are still not always put together, optimized, and crystal clear, but rather, complex, dynamic, and full spectrum. Yet, through it all, they keep on shining.

The difference between someone staying stuck or thriving is simply the choice to continuously evolve, like a Phoenix rising from the ashes. They adapt, overcome, uplevel, and do the work to take responsibility for their lives. They take their power back, they set boundaries, they accept, they heal, and they continue to stay openhearted. They rise in gratitude proclaiming everything has been for them to learn and to grow, all for their highest good. People who radiate an inner beauty have known loss, have been defeated, experienced deep suffering, and have found a way out of the depths and into the light. Being a soulful person doesn't happen by accident. We are stretched and expanded through adversity. The most resilient of us are forged in the fire. Remember, the powerful Phoenix rises from the ashes, not from rainbows and waterfalls.

Life's difficulties are universal, although often unevenly distributed. Whether from marginalized communities or bearing generational traumas, many are trapped in cycles of deep suffering. Yet we're all descendants of survivors—Ancestors—who weathered natural disasters, wars, and pandemics. If you dig deep within yourself, you may discover lingering feelings of anxiety, fear, or even numbness and indifference. These emotions are often signs of unaddressed pain.

Also, everyone living in a post-colonization, capitalistic, monarchy, dictatorship, or any other patriarchal form of governed society is inevitably traumatized after decades of bypassing and perpetuating the corruption and destruction inherent to these systems. The impacts of society will get to you eventually, and the pain that comes with unconscious ways of being will bring you into the furnace. But instead of anger, bitterness, rage, or resentment burning you from the inside out, allow life to stoke your fire—a fire that is tended to with curiosity and compassion can, and will, change the world. All your feelings must be felt for life to be lived to the fullest.

I invite you to check in with yourself, in this moment, in order to make space for the beauty and the blessings, and see if there is anything that needs to be transmuted in the fire. Are there parts that have to die so that you can be born again? Check in with what is on your heart. Are there any past hurts, mistakes, and regrets that you have? Do you feel anxious instead of excited? Do you feel scared instead of secure? Feel into the full spectrum, both the positive and the negative, the heavy and the hopeful, and try to do so without preference or judgment. Witness it all, feel it all, become it all, and receive the gift life holds for you when you explore the darkness and feel the heat.

There may be things, memories, or hurts you discover that you may have forgotten or thought maybe weren't a big deal. Get a journal to keep record of what those things are. You can let this be a stepping stone to new life. Write them, read them aloud, feel them, bring them into the light of pure presence, and in your own time, notice if there is an emotional charge that still surrounds it. If so, let it inform, motivate, and remind you. Where do you feel sensations alive in your body? What does it look like or feel like? Is it soft or hard, round or edged, colorful or dark? Remember, you are always safe being in the present moment. Breathe deep into your belly, let the exhale be longer than the inhale, let tears come if they come, and then notice if the charge dissipates.

We must die a million deaths to become who we are meant to be. To access our light at full brilliance, it takes plunging into the depths of darkness. Like the Phoenix, we dive into the flames and are reborn through the process of transformation. We will do this many times if we allow ourselves, whether we are aware that it's happening or not. Learning to become aware and conscious of this process is the key to living a truly fulfilled life. While dying unto ourselves can seem scary and full of suffering, it is a blessing to be reborn because it implies growth and evolution. Experiencing countless deaths while we are still alive is a natural and critical part of life. Moment to moment, day to day, lifetime to lifetime, we live, we die, we are renewed, and we get to do it again and again.

We are here to shine. After every little death, we renew, and we live on. We have work to do, but it is divine work. It isn't only sunshine and rainbows on this path of remembering your roots. It is diving deep into the soil, integrating what awaits us in the darkness, letting life inform us, nourish us, and empower us. Those of us who have been through the fire are trail blazers, here to light up the path for a brighter future for all. As you do this type of spiritual work, you may feel as if you are a healer of yourself, your lineage, and maybe of the world. What you truly are is someone who is simply participating in the healing process. Healing happens. It's not something you make happen, just as you don't make a plant grow. What you are wise to do is give yourself and others the essential and optimal conditions for growth, for healing, and for the emergence of gratitude to simply happen. And like a plant, the further you reach your roots into the darkness, the higher you reach to the life-giving fire in the sky.

You are here for full-spectrum aliveness. You are not here to be a perfect angel or a pedestaled guru. What we need is more authenticity, loyalty to the raw and imperfect, and an honor of the light and the dark that lives within all of us.

## *Conclusion*

My Mayan elders believe that each element offers an essential cleansing and that the elements are here to remind us of what's true. The waters cleanse our body, the winds clear our mind, yet the fire is the only element that can clear away the energetic body, your aura, and your DNA. They believe there is a lot for us to cleanse—residue we've built up within our bodies from our own lifetime or from our lineage. We must turn to the simple but essential wisdom of the water, the earth, and the air.

Within our DNA, we have things to be burned away that we've compiled.

Mayan shamanism is centered around fire ceremonies. In ceremonies, they count the days, offer their prayers, offerings, and gratitude, and also cleanse the energies within themselves, each other, their community, and the world. One of my Mayan teachers and spiritual guides, Nana Lu, an Aj Q'ij and fire keeper, shared with me that the fire is considered "the ear of God" to the Maya because God can hear our prayers through the fire. Through this element, we can learn to listen to the primordial, life-giving wisdom and messages that God has for us. When we come to the fire with questions, the fire will speak to the Aj Q'ij, and they will share the ways the fire has spoken. They will give advice on how to tend to life's obstacles and sometimes give you rituals and guidance to follow in order to support your journey.

A practical and powerful tool can be found by looking to our animal kin for guidance. Wild animals do not hold on to trauma. Instead, they shake to release any built-up energy. When an animal has experienced a high level of stress, they will shake it out, vocalize, and move on. We are really not so different than animals, and when we move and shake our bodies, we release pent-up energy as well. Dogs often shake themselves after a stressful or highly stimulating event as a way to reset. If a spider monkey was just hunted by a jaguar, and it escaped, after the chase and finding a safe place, he'll let everyone in the neighborhood know what just happened with an unashamed, piercing cry that echoes throughout the jungle. A male goose will also shake his wings violently after a conflict with another goose to release his stress. Only after clearing the energy do these animals go about their day.

Since I used to not feel safe expressing my feelings, I pleased and appeased, distracting myself from my natural suffering. But now, I let the intelligence of nature flow through me. After a difficult, triggering, or intense experience, mimicking my wise animal Ancestors, I shake it out, yell, hit or scream into a pillow, stomp my feet, have a tantrum, curse, and let my feelings move without directing that energy toward anyone else. The spider monkey is not mad at the jaguar, and its cries are not blaming, shaming, or projecting. The monkey uses its voice, moves its body, and goes into a healthy fight-or-flight response to cope with stress. We, too, can use our voice and physical movement as outlets for stress, without directing negative energy toward others.

We are so much more than our experiences, more than our thoughts, more than our emotions. Yet our feelings must be validated, spoken, felt, and expressed in a healthy way. When we feel safe and ready, we must express these emotions. This means practicing letting your body express without having to have words by shaking, walking, running, yelling (in a comfortable space), singing, dancing, and whatever allows you to come into harmony and feel safe in your body. Only then are we fully alive; only then do we allow the flames to fuel us. We must respect the sacred fire. If not, we will scar our hearts from the heat of misplaced rage, unreleased passion, or stifled love.

Reach for the skies, and allow the fire of the sun to warm your leaves. Reach deep into the fiery core of the Earth, your roots so deep, so secure, so alive that you can't help but thrive.

### *Embodiment Practice: Rage Ritual*

This ritual can be used at the peak of feeling anger so you can channel and direct your energy in a way that supports you rather than burns you up. You must engage consciously with intense emotions, or they will leak out in ways equally as destructive as major, volcanic explosions. You can do this practice even if you don't feel upset about anything specific. Really, this practice is best done when feeling generally okay, grounded, and settled within yourself. That way, you're able to dive beneath the surface and feel into the depths of your fiery soul without getting overwhelmed.

Begin by becoming aware of your feelings, whatever they may be in the moment. Close your eyes. Take six deep breaths in through the nose and out through the mouth. Feel your body relax and open. Put on music that will help you feel more deeply whatever is presently on your heart. If feeling some anger, put on a song with heavy drums or something that puts you into a more-intense-than-normal state. Begin shaking your whole body first, bouncing up and down and gently flailing arms and hands. Shaking is so good for your health. It helps let go of stress and anxiety, it stimulates the lymphatic system, it boosts the immune system, and it activates relaxation in the body. After shaking for at least a few minutes without stopping, pause and check in with how you feel. Do you feel you made some space? Do you feel less in your head? Do you feel silly? Do you feel lightened? Shake until you feel yourself shift your state of being.

Next, if you're feeling a deeper sense of rage, try hitting a pillow. Do this carefully to protect your back and neck. I recommend kneeling on your bed, keeping your back and arms straight, putting one of your fists into the other hand, and beating the pillow with the back of your fists and your forearms. You don't have to destroy it and beat it to smithereens. Do it just enough to feel yourself really getting out of your normal mindset and into the new territory of expressing your feelings. Use your voice to grunt, growl, or scream as you hit the pillow or stomp on the floor. Make sure to yell from your core and deep from your belly so you do not strain your voice. Let your body move with the anger as if it were moving through and out of you. Remember, when we let go of these blockages that keep us contained, we accept our darkness, rage, and anger which gives space for new light to shine through. There's no reason to shame ourselves for these feelings. They are not us. Emotions are just energy in motion that needs to be expressed. Remember, you are the source of light, and all energy can enhance the light that shines from you!

If in this process you feel grief, put on a song that stirs those emotions. Let yourself feel sadness. If you don't feel comfortable moving your body, close your eyes and rock back and forth until you begin moving dynamically, free of thoughts or judgments. Simply feel the music and feel your heart. Let the body move as it wants to. The body has its own intelligence, so allow it to do what it wants. You may realize your arms begin to unfurl and float, your hips begin to sway, and it may start to feel really good and different than what you're used to. Whatever you feel is perfect. Only after feeling and moving through grief, will we have space to truly feel gratitude, pleasure, and celebration.

When you're ready to feel deep gratitude, put on a feel-good song like "Dog Days Are Over" by Florence and the Machine or whatever makes you feel free! Then, transition into a gratitude dance. When you begin with this dance, allow gratitude to be felt in your heart, first and foremost. Imagine gratitude as a feeling of warmth like a fire, like the sun in the center of your radiant heart, and then let that light spread throughout your entire being. Use your imagination to imagine how you would feel if you were truly grateful. What would your life look like to be filled with bliss, joy, and pleasure? What would it feel like? Taste like? Smell like? Come into the sensations of feeling gratitude! Let your body move as freely as it would like to. Let your body become the embodiment of gratitude through your unique expression, celebrating the simple joy of dancing!

CHAPTER 9:

# Surrendering to the Flow

*"In one drop of water are found all the secrets of all the oceans; in one aspect of you are found all the aspects of existence."*

— Kahlil Gibran

Life on this planet began when asteroids impacted water that covered the surface of the Earth. This union of fire and water laid the blueprint from which all life as we know evolved. As I shared, fire is the purest essence of the Creator and creation. Therefore, fire is the spark of the soul, and water is the host for life to emerge, just like the womb of a pregnant mother. When this flaming ball of energy entered into the Earth's watery womb, there was an explosion of potential life. When you combine fire and water, much like when volcanic magma runs into the ocean, rain falls upon lava, or a sperm and egg unite, something new is created. Our human body, just like the planet, is a creation of the primordial elements of fire and water in perfect harmony.

Being in flow is our original state of being. As we evolve in the womb as an embryo, first and foremost, we are a water-based organism. In this developing state, life is a mystery. We are semiconscious, for we respond to touch, sound, and our mother's environment. In the water, our mothers' blood, nutrients, and emotional nourishment combine with the light of our unique and immortal, undying soul. This process is what makes us who we are in this lifetime. Only after the "water breaks" and the birth process begins, just like life evolving from ocean to land, do we also leave the primordial habitat of water and enter the world as we now know it.

All things are living because of water, and water itself must be alive for it to give life in return. If water is stagnant, it becomes a breeding ground for bacteria, pathogens, and forms of life that are dangerous to our health. If you observe cats, who are an ancient and mysterious species themselves, they rarely drink still water. Certain kinds of cats will drink water out of a dirty toilet bowl as it's flushing before they drink still, lifeless water out of a bowl. This is very curious indeed, and we are wise to learn that moving water is best, but unlike our feline friends, we'll definitely stick to drinking out of cups, or from anything we can give our water a solid swirl before ingesting.

When water moves, especially in a circular motion, it comes to life! Water is known as $H_2O$, which means it's made of two hydrogen atoms to every one oxygen atom. One hydrogen atom and the oxygen atom are constantly bonded, but the extra hydrogen atom gets exchanged between different $H_2O$ molecules. When water is in motion, the rate that the extra hydrogen atom is exchanged speeds up. It's like the water turns into a completely different state, one that's dynamic and quantum. Stagnant water means that there is not enough energy to exchange that extra hydrogen between molecules. That's why I said to give your water a swirl before you drink it. The motion speeds up the exchange of the extra hydrogen atom and brings your water more to life.

### *Active Surrender*

The opposite of flow is stagnation, which comes from fear, shutting down, and not trusting. For example, we often fear something bad will happen. This places us in a prolonged "freeze" trauma response, which is another form of stagnation. When water is frozen, there is no passing of the extra hydrogen atom, thus it is lifeless. When we go into a freeze response, we too are without life. Therefore, to shift into trust and into flow, which is our natural state of being, you must be able to dive below the surface and get in touch with your deeper feelings.

When I was around the age of 12, my mom let me bring my best friend on a trip to Big Bear, California. At night, we lit a fire in the cabin's fireplace and went to bed. The fire grew as we slept, burning outside of the fireplace and engulfing the entire living room. I will never forget my mother running into our bedroom in a panic, yelling at us to get up and run. I was ready to flee, but my best friend froze and curled up into a ball. Her response to trauma was freezing.

If you have the tendency to freeze under stress, you want to keep your inner fire alive to find a different response. When we are under stress, our bodies naturally need to move. Even if a wild animal freezes for a moment from headlights or another shock to their nervous system, once they move forward, they'll shake vigorously to release the trauma. Dogs do this when they're startled too.

Zebras and antelope do this if they survive close calls with a predator. It's important to accept that sometimes we may need to bare our teeth like a jaguar rather than get frozen like deer in headlights.

The ideal state of body and mind is what I call "active surrender." This means holding strong boundaries like the banks of a river, so the natural flow of water can stay active and stay alive. If there were no banks to a river, it would become a pond or lake. It's the boundaries that keep the water flowing along, and you are no different. Only when you have strong boundaries can you surrender to the flow. If someone from your past or present demolishes your boundaries, or pressures you, you may go into a freeze trauma response. Another way to cope is to divert your course and break your flow by people pleasing to avoid conflict. This is a fawn trauma response. While it's natural to resort to these instinctual behaviors, it's more beneficial to transcend these basic impulses. If you need to fight or flee, channel your powerful inner waters, but make sure you utilize the practices from the last chapter as well as what you will learn in this one to come back into balance.

The best option is to confidently stay your course, maintain clear boundaries, and focus only on being in flow—those who are meant to join, expand, and enliven your flow will find you, and you will find them. Trust yourself. Be like water. Rage, crash, drizzle, or deluge as you feel is necessary. Tap into the power of this primordial element, but don't become frozen or stay stagnant in life. Remember, water carries all the information from all life, so trust the waters that flow within the blood in your body.

### *Beauty Is in the Depths*

Evolutionarily, since we all came from the water, being in flow is how we feel most fully alive. In previous chapters, you have made space for healing by understanding your triggers, integrating negative emotions, and expressing rage healthfully. You've walked through the fires and have emerged reborn. The most beautiful people are those who return to the fires and give water to those still in the heat of it. However, it's no small thing to dive below the surface and find what lurks in the darkness of deep water. But when you do, what you find isn't as scary as you think it is. Just like going into the vast ocean, the emotions associated with water like sadness, depression, and grief can feel heavy and dark. So, instead of riding the waves, it often seems more peaceful to lounge on the beach and bask in the sunshine. If you do venture into the water, it can truly be a religious experience. Not only because of the danger of drowning, but because it's like reentering the womb, the womb of your First Mother, the holder of all life's records, and home of the Great Mystery.

One of Syris's core childhood memories was one of the first times he was in the ocean. He was around eight years old in Outer Banks, North Carolina. The waves were much bigger than what he was used to closer to home at Virginia Beach, yet unsurprisingly, he went out a bit farther than he should have into some of the bigger surf. Quickly, he got caught in a series of big waves. No one was there to see his predicament, nor was he taught how to either "duck-dive" underneath or ride the waves as they came. He was put in a spin cycle, fighting and struggling to reach the surface, but the waves kept coming. Just before he really began drowning, a family friend ran over and pulled him to the surface. This was Syris's first experience with active surrender, and it stands as one of the most formative moments of his entire life.

He learned that day to ride the waves of life, and when big waves come crashing, much like big feelings, to do what seems like the last thing someone should do. The most simple yet courageous choice is to dive right into it. Now, one of Syris's favorite places in the entire world is to be directly underneath a wave. It's quiet and still, yet it's a symphony of Nature's raw power. Here, he feels himself being reminded of who he, and we all, truly are. Instead of getting caught up in the drama and trauma of heavy emotions, you can stay afloat and ride the waves, or dive underneath the surface.

It can be scary to face our fears and feel our feelings. Every instinct tells us "escape" or "fight." But when in water, or during deep feelings, the only way to survive, and be fully alive, is to surrender to the flow and dive right in. While both anxiety and excitement are the same to the body, it's the mind that knows the difference. Anxiety usually stems from fear of the unknown or possible negative consequences, whereas excitement is a positive anticipation of what's to come. If you feel anxiety, you can shift it to excitement by consciously changing your perspective, signaling to your body that you're actually eager for the opportunities that the unknown may bring.

Depression is another deep emotional state. Depression can be the result of being exhausted from fighting to stay afloat and keep up a certain identity or persona. If you've been depressed, you know it feels like you're sinking to the bottom of the ocean or are being forcibly pulled down. Here, it's easy to believe that nothing or no one can fix us . . . and that's true. If something is broken, in a mechanistic worldview, then it's true that broken things need fixing. However, people don't need fixing, because no one is fundamentally broken. In a holistic worldview, we are perfectly imperfect, and simply out of balance. However, if we identify with our mind or body, then there is always something telling us we need to be different or better. What we need is to love ourselves and to have others in our life who accept us being our true selves. Only then can we drop all the masks that block us shining as our powerful, radiant self. Self-love and community are the two ultimate antidotes to depression.

One of the most dynamic feelings that lurks in the deep is grief. Grief is commonly known to have five defined stages, but for me, these come in waves and happen in their own time. These five known aspects are denial, anger, bargaining, depression, and acceptance. One of the unspoken parts of grief is relief. After Syris's mother endured a yearlong battle with leukemia, once she passed, there was a surprising sense of relief that came along with all the other stages of grief. Even if one of these stages isn't felt, let's say bargaining, it's helpful to dive into it and feel your way through it. Or, if you're unable to feel any sense of relief or that any good can come from such hard, intense, or tragic events, just imagine what relief would feel like. Plunge headfirst into the ocean of remembrance, even, and especially, if that means you'll find grief in the depths. Allow yourself to receive the wisdom that awaits you under the surface of everyday, routine living.

There is no right way to grieve, but major issues can ensue if you do not grieve. While it is common to hold on to the past or resist a pain in your present reality, especially after a death, tragedy, or intense experience, all it does is block the natural flow of life. To experience the full depth of gratitude, it's essential to fully acknowledge and grieve life's losses and challenges. Gratitude is our most alive and vital state of being. As long as we are alive, we'll navigate between the contrasting yet connected experiences of grief and gratitude, each one enriching the depth and fullness of the other.

The place that is most activated when we feel the depths of our feelings is the heart. Our hearts will flow between opening and closing. We heal our hearts so that we can remain open and keep loving, ensuring that life force energy continues to flow throughout our bodies. Unlike what Western religions tell us, our hearts are wise beyond measure. We can and must trust our hearts. However, we must not mistake the limited desires of the mind for the loving desires of the heart.

We also must honor and worship the sacred waters that flow within us. And we must live in complete reverence for when these inner waters show themselves externally through bleeding, sweating, and crying. For women, our blood each month is an offering back to the soil. We all, but men especially, must release their tears and sweat to cleanse their emotions through their bodies. For thousands of years, women have been crying from the pain of imbalances seen through relational, emotional, physical, and systemic abuse. When men finally feel their feelings, dive to the depths of their own inner darkness, and express it, they will heal fully and there will be a fundamental shift on every level of life on the planet.

Tears come when the heart is activated through grief or gratitude. On a hormonal level, certain chemicals are released when we cry. Suppressing an emotion heightens pain and makes you feel worse. So, while you might think you're soothing yourself by not crying, stress is actually intensifying. Resisting crying in the short-term can cause problems such as irritability, anxiety, and poor sleep. But over time, repressing your tears can lead to diseases of the heart such as hypertension or even cancer. Tears are our sacred waters, cleansing us like only sacred water can.

### *God Is in the Water*

In ancient times, it is theorized that instead of libraries, inhabitants of Atlantis had great bowls from which people would drink water, hold it in their mouth, access divine knowledge, and then spit back into these great bowls. When someone wanted to "read the book" or receive the knowledge, they would simply drink from the bowl containing all the information people passed into it. While this may seem highly infectious and unbelievable, it proposes a curious idea: that water holds memory and can store information.

If water truly covered the face of the planet, for it is simply an evolved state of hydrogen and oxygen, and it existed before any life was created, then, since the very first forms of life formed within the waters, it holds memory from the first spark of life to the world as we know it today. While there is no modern scientific proof of this, Indigenous cultures believe that water holds, stores, and retains the entire record of all evolution of life. It carries ancient information, and it also hydrates us, plants, and animals, giving us the ability to continue living. Therefore, for Atlanteans, to record all their own history by adding the waters of their body through their saliva to the waters of the world, they were simply adding their own data into Nature's information storage system.

Water is the single most important element for living things. Water gives and sustains life and is the home in which life is born. We drink it, bathe in it, and swim in it, and it flows within us. Water is the ultimate shapeshifter and interacts with gravitational forces in unique ways, seemingly defying the laws of gravity due to its special properties. The human body is about 60 percent water by weight, and molecularly, it's around 99 percent water. This means you are primarily made up of the most ancient and vital substance in the universe. Our survival relies on fresh, clean, and living water. Moreover, studies prove that water responds to human emotion and amplifies our prayers and intentions. Like all the elements—and like each of us—water possesses its own kind of magic. We can see that, like water, we can be stagnant or living in flow. Do you feel you are able to move with the waves of life, or do you get easily stagnant or sluggish when you are uncomfortable? When you are triggered, do you freeze up, or can you flow boldly? Pause and feel the rhythm of your heartbeat and the water of your blood flowing through you, giving life to every cell of your body.

To truly support a life lived in flow, it is critical to have access to clean, chemical-free water, and to drink plenty of it. Water is sacred, and to live fully, we must honor it with the utmost gratitude. I used to be chronically dehydrated, always trying to catch up on drinking enough water. I also used to have painful periods with spotty bleeds. As soon as I started drinking over three liters a day, my moon cycle was healthier and easier. Since I was finally hydrated, I'd bleed a healthy, natural crimson red color each day of my period. This means I was clearing out my womb, and now I have little to no cramps or pain. When we give ourselves enough water, it hydrates all our cells and allows our body to naturally cleanse, release, and make space for life to flow through us.

Remember that water is life. Water is cleansing. Water is sacred. Humans all over the world use water to cleanse themselves both physically as well as energetically. Water has its own intelligence and memory just like all living things do. Water, our planet's most vital element, is the link that binds all forms of life together. It nourishes us, moves within and around us, and renews our bodies. Serving as Earth's lifeblood, water purifies both the planet and all its inhabitants. Its various manifestations—rivers, lakes, ice, and oceans—are essential to the well-being of both our planet and ourselves. The diverse forms and functions of water, including the homes it provides for countless creatures, contribute to the overall health and vitality of all that exist outside its depths.

Water's sacred nature instructs us that we can possess immense power, enough to reshape even towering mountains, while remaining gentle, yielding, and adaptable. It symbolizes that, like water, our life's journey also has no real beginning nor end; one day the river of our life will run into the ocean, rejoining with the Great Mystery from which we came.

### *Embodiment Practice: Water Work*

You can work directly with water to cultivate a lifestyle of flow. You can do this in simple or ceremonial ways. Your shower at morning or night is a place for deep cleansing, receiving new insights, setting intentions, and refreshing yourself from the outside in and the inside out.

Like ancient cultures have and still do, you can sing or speak prayers, intentions, or affirmations into your water, and all liquids, before drinking it. Since water holds memory and is the record of life, by using your voice to infuse your water with loving intentions, when you drink it, you will become the living embodiment of those prayers.

Also, I invite you to go to a natural body of water like the ocean, a river, or natural spring. Make it a self-love date or a time to connect with others. Remember, self-love and community are the antidotes to any kind of mental or emotional suffering, and there is no better place to find healing than in the waters of our First Mother. Give thanks to the water for its cleansing and purifying properties, and then enter fully into the water with the intention of washing away all the thoughts or past stories you'd like to let go of. Feel yourself free from all the residue you've released, and come out of the water feeling refreshed, renewed, and reborn.

CHAPTER 10:

# THE BREATH OF LIFE

*"Magic is everywhere; as natural a part of our world as the air we breathe."*

— PAULO COELHO

We can be sure of two things throughout our life: that we are meant to evolve, and that our breath will remain with us until we depart this world. If we stay in our comfort zone and attempt to remain the same, we will not accept that change is inevitable, necessary, and beneficial. When we embrace and surrender to change, growth happens. If we insist on fighting the natural order of things, we will harden our mind, body, and heart, causing disease and premature death. Although change can feel scary and uncomfortable, by embracing discomfort and leaning in to things that challenge us, we find our resiliency and strength. This is how we learn more about who we truly are and what makes us unique.

Change is hard and messy, like the caterpillar that turns into a sludgy mess in the darkness of its own cocoon.

Yet this transformation is sprinkled with some mysterious magic that allows it to morph into a butterfly. It's the same for us. When we embrace our own shadows and those cast by others, and surrender to change instead of resisting, we uncover and evolve into more wondrous versions of ourselves. When we surrender to the magic of change, we transform. Through that process, we alchemize the past versions of ourselves and become renewed in the process.

To make true growth and evolve in a beautiful way, we must make peace with the past. Many of our ailments, illnesses, and troubles stem from living stuck in the past, even if we are not aware that we're doing so. When we stay stuck in past hardships or are anxious about the future, we give our power away. When we release the past and learn to have faith for the future, we reclaim our power. When we forgive, we're extending compassion to those who hurt us—and that includes ourselves. This brings us into reality, into the present moment, grateful to be here now. We no longer hold on to a past version of ourselves or others, because in this moment, we are entirely different beings than who we were a week ago, a month ago, years past, or even just yesterday. We can change, heal, and move forward, closer to our true selves with the smallest of steps. Sometimes it takes finding ourselves at rock bottom to realize this, like I was, or we can learn from the past and make changes right now.

You do not have to get to rock bottom to make changes or have life-altering realizations. You can learn from my story and others; that is why we are here with and for each other. I share my story because I know there are people just like me, who felt how I did, and struggled to make a change. I will never forget when I finally decided to lean in to and accept change. At my life's rock bottom, I stepped fully into the discomfort of change because staying comfortable with an abusive, toxic partner was more painful than the unknown. In that way, a bad relationship can remind us how everything happens for us, to teach us something, and direct us into the evolution of our soul. We may not see it that way when we're in the thick of it, but looking back on challenging experiences, you can find that you learned something from them. Ultimately, the goal is to find gratitude for the fact that you are here now because of anything and everything you went through. Doing so, you claim your power instead of leaving it in the hands of the people, places, and experiences that challenged you.

At my rock bottom, I wasn't aware of it at the time, but I was replaying a pattern so I could break free from it. I was experiencing another toxic environment that was just like the one I experienced in my childhood that also led me to feel hopeless and confused. I could have stayed in that and died slowly as I was, or I could change my life and live fully. The Universe was saying, "Are you listening? Are you paying attention? Would you like to evolve? Yes? Okay, great! Start by remembering your inherent worth. You are so much more than this. You are expansive, infinite potential, unconditional love, divinity, and the embodiment of magic. Remember who you truly are, dearly beloved."

So, I stood up, choosing to live and evolve. I said thank you to the Universe for the lesson and moved forward toward alignment and contentment, one step at a time. It started with small changes like taking a yoga class, reading spiritual books like Louise Hay's *You Can Heal Your Life* (by a magical twist of fate, this book has been published by Hay House), drinking relaxing herbal teas, listening to Oprah's *Super Soul Sunday*, meditating, doing breathwork, exploring foreign countries, and experiencing different ways of living. Keeping an open mind allowed me to slowly open my heart. These actions led me down the path to discover that I could change and that my life truly had purpose.

Our small choices add up to big changes. *Change* is a funny word; what we experience is more like an *unfurling*. When we evolve, we are becoming more of our true self. More of our soul is able to shine through, which has always been there, but now we are able to be free and express ourselves more authentically. It takes willingness and openness to allow the path back to yourself to unfold before you. But often, the process of unfurling can feel like it's too much.

When this happens, come back to the breath. Your breath is your companion for your entire lifetime. It is your anchor to the present moment. It is the only thing you control, moment to moment, that keeps you alive. Whenever you're feeling ungrounded, anxious, or purposeless, return to your breath. Your breath is your most powerful tool to live a better, brighter, and healthier life.

Learn to lean in to the sweetness of a slow and deep inhale and an even slower exhalation when change is happening. Breathing slowly in through your nose and slowly out through your mouth is cleansing to your nervous system. You can also practice "box breath," a potent breathing technique to ground your body and mind. I do the box breath before I sleep, and Syris was trained during his Air Force Special Operations training to do this to relax his nervous system. So, if it worked for him with the stress he was under, you know it works well. The way it works is you inhale for five seconds, hold your breath for five seconds, exhale for five seconds, and then hold for five seconds. You can do a few rounds of this before coming back to normal breathing. I visualize my whole body relaxing when I exhale. My jaw unhinges, my lips soften, my eyes roll back, my forehead relaxes, and the back of my head melts into the surface beneath me. Doing this, I always feel myself surrender to deep relaxation.

You can also use breath to energize yourself. Any time you breathe in with your mouth, you are "up-regulating" your nervous system. This is why you want to make sure you breathe in and out through your nose while you sleep to maximize your rest and restoration. But if you are feeling groggy, sluggish, or static in your energy, some quick breaths in and out of your mouth can change your state. I like to do this instead of turning to caffeine or other stimulants. Our body is so intelligent, and we are wise to tap into the simple but effective ways of energizing or calming ourselves, all through the oxygen that Mother Nature so abundantly provides.

### *Breathing into Your True Self*

If we do not make a shift from within, we will continue to see the same patterns show up in our outer world. Our external environment reflects our inner garden. However, we all have things we are unaware of, and we cannot know them until they are reflected to us. These triggers invite us to shift out of the pattern, explore its roots, and then evolve into a deeper connection with ourselves, others, and our reality. Doing this work, we will gain a felt understanding, a gnosis, and make peace with all parts of ourselves. This is why it is essential to reprogram our minds so that we break free from old patterns. We are quick learners, but it takes practice, it takes discipline, and it takes devotion to our highest self. And yes, the lessons, triggers, and patterns may come back again, but you have the tools from this book to use when you are being tested. Remember your breath—a tool that's ever available, ready to guide you fully into your purpose, and is happening every single moment. Become aware of your breath, and you will become aware of everything you are.

Living life in awareness is not the easiest thing to do. Likewise, it isn't easy to stay unaware and numb to life either. Living isn't about choosing easy. Living takes work. The gift in becoming more aware is that once you remember who you are, you start to remember why you are here. You remember that you are meant to evolve, grow, and love through all experiences, whether they're challenging or not. Once you start to do the work to remember your roots, by practicing gratitude, it gets easier and easier to live in awareness of both the hard things and the blissful things. Being aware does not mean life will be perfect from here on out. It means that you will be in the driver's seat, the empowered creator of your entire reality, and that you will be able to follow the thread of gratitude back to your heart even when you are hurting.

Any attempt at finding acceptance or love outside of yourself is futile, for humans often disappoint if you give your power away to them. What we do instead is look to our True Self for guidance. The True Self is one with Spirit; it is connected to the Cosmos, Mother Nature, the loving Ancestors, and guides. It's the part of you that knows who you really are, what you need to do in any given moment, and it's that felt sense of clearheaded confidence. Accessing our intention and attention, we can remember our True Self with a single breath. Seek your True Self if ever you think anyone else has the answers or has it better than you. The True Self is who you are underneath all the programs you have taken on and mistaken yourself as.

When we access our higher self, our True Self, we will live a life of purpose. We are each here for a unique purpose. Sometimes we know what that is. Other times it changes, shifts, and evolves, or goes away completely. Whether you feel like you know your purpose right now or not, remember to remain connected to your breath, and you will be led exactly where you need to go. When you identify your karma, develop your persona, and live in a state of gratitude, your dharma will unfurl before you like magic.

I followed the nudges of my heart, taking little steps at a time that led me to find my purpose. I traveled the world, discovering yoga and then cacao, which helped me open my heart, claim my truth, and access my magic. In the beginning of your journey, you're not supposed to immediately know what your purpose is. Remember that that's okay. Follow your heart and trust your bliss, because what lights you up is an indicator that you are following your purpose. Also, your purpose doesn't have to be how you generate income. But a great idea is that your vocation should be where your own personal passions meet the greatest need you're able to support with.

Having difficult conversations, loving others, accepting loss, and moving through difficulties are key actions to finding our True Self. When you want to go deeper, you can get assistance from professionals, elders, and mentors. You can also look further out to the stars to see that your personality, your strengths, and weaknesses are also written in the Cosmos awaiting your recognition. The sacred Mayan Calendar is one of the ways in which you can learn more about yourself, using its knowledge to inform you of your purpose. You can also make a list in your journal of things that light you up. Just write the first things that come to mind. Review your list and number them from most to least exciting. For each of the things listed, write two things you're already doing related to it and then list three things you can start doing to make it fully become your reality. This will allow you to work toward knowing the ins and outs of how you can shift into living your purpose fully.

Following my purpose started with believing I was meant to share cacao with the world. My purpose now includes many things, but in the beginning, I dedicated my time to learning all I needed to learn about cacao, simply because it lit me up. It excited me to learn about my ancestral plant and connect with my roots, lineage, and magic. The more you follow your bliss, the more the path expands before you. When you listen to the wisdom of the winds and are flowing like a river, eventually it leads to a crystalline lake or an ocean of possibilities. When you're in flow, it leads you straight to magic.

### *The Wisdom of the Wind*

The wind is a mysterious element. It can bring pleasant smells and just as quickly take them away. It carries the voice of someone we love, the songs of a bird, the laugh of a baby, and the salt of the sea. The wind can whip, leaving us feeling ungrounded if we're imbalanced, or it can guide us to places we wouldn't have known without it. The wind whispers and it howls. It beckons and it directs. It kicks up leaves, blows hair in our face, and dances with the trees. We can ride its drafts up to great heights, seeing life from a new perspective. Then, we could be caught in a sandstorm, get sand in our eyes, not even able to see two steps in front of us. The wind is ever-changing, yet it always brings an invitation for us to be fully present.

Feel your breath as the same breath of your First Mother. Listen to what the wind whispers and remind yourself that if you get caught in a storm, to never panic but remember, you don't always have to see the whole picture. Most of the time, all you need is to see the next step in front of you. And if you can't even see that, take a deep breath, and take the next best step anyway.

The Maya believe that words are extremely powerful and that we should only speak words of truth with sweetness and kindness. Whatever words you say are heard, picked up, and carried by the wind to all ends of the planet. Whatever you say, it will return to you tenfold. So, speak with intention, playfulness, and with wisdom. Send your prayers out into the wind, knowing that it will touch exactly who it's meant to. Trust the wind, feel its guidance, and if you ever feel ungrounded, simply take another breath. Feeling grounded, guided, present, and on-purpose, in this moment, breathe gratitude into every area of your life.

*"Breathing in, I am aware of my heart.*
*Breathing out, I smile to my heart [ . . . ].*
*I feel grateful for my heart."*

— Khalil Gibran

### *Embodiment Practice: Gratitude Breathwork*

For this Gratitude Breathwork practice, sit up nice and tall with your hands on your knees. Close your eyes. Relax your forehead, eyes, the back of your head, mouth, tongue, jaw, and neck. Feel your whole body is relaxed; belly soft and relaxed. Inhale into your belly and exhale, relaxing further. Feel your body being filled with breath.

With your next inhale, breathe in love, and on the exhale, breathe out gratitude. Say to yourself or aloud, while you inhale, "I am awareness, breathing in love," and while you exhale, "I am awareness, breathing out gratitude."

See if you can imagine a loving light entering through you from the top of your head as you inhale, and see that light exit down through your feet, into the soil and all around you. Do this a few times, and once you truly feel yourself overflowing with love and gratitude, place your hand on your heart. Return to your natural breath and with your radiant heart. Give thanks. Maltyox.

As mentioned in the chapter, breathwork is a dynamic tool to use every day, as much as you can remember throughout the day. Box breathing can be used to down-regulate, while heavy mouth breathing can be used to energize, or up-regulate. I also like to meditate and do breathwork outdoors. Feel the difference, the subtlety between the wind contacting your face and your own breath going in your nose. Focus solely on the intake of air passing over the top of your lip and into the tip of your nose. It's an isolated place to put your full awareness, an anchor, that brings you fully into the moment.

CHAPTER 11:

# Shadows and Sunshine

*"The healing of our present woundedness may lie in recognizing and reclaiming the capacity we all have to heal each other."*

— Yung Pueblo

Distraction is the only way many of us know how to cope with big feelings. It is not only accepted but widely advertised to avoid difficult feelings like anger, sadness, or grief. We live in a society that pretends emotions don't exist by drinking, eating, sleeping, medicating, or smoking them away, suppressing our feelings as quickly and efficiently as possible. What we as individuals and the whole of humanity need most are safe spaces to feel the full range of our emotions. What we all need are more ceremonies in our life. In a ceremony, we have the opportunity to become fully present so we can connect with and heal our body, mind, and soul. When we are intentional and create a sacred space, our healing work is amplified. This is the power of ceremony.

Ceremony is a defining aspect of Indigenous cultures all over the world, and it is an intentional space to commune with and give thanks to the unseen worlds, realms, and forces of good. In a ceremony, you have the opportunity to feel a sense of deep reverence, gratitude, honor, and remembrance. This is a time to give thanks to all that is, connect with pure energies, communicate with God, release that which no longer serves, manifest a new reality, and honor the process of life. A rite of passage, like a birthday, death, and birth are ceremonies each of us have and will experience. By consciously engaging in ceremony, we reclaim our roots and tap into the wise ways of our ancient Ancestors.

No matter your background, all our Ancestors performed ceremonies. For some of our lineages, these practices were taken away to keep them from accessing a direct connection to God and Creator without a church or someone else being an intermediary. When we reclaim ceremony, we infuse the sacred into our lives, reclaiming our ancestral ways and powerful practices to live grounded and rooted into the true nature of life. When we know, have, and develop our own relationship with God, we realize that we can infuse the sacred into everything we do and make our life a continuous ceremony.

I didn't know what a ceremony truly was until I went to Bali many years ago. By witnessing the Balinese people, I realized for the first time how prevalent sacred ceremonies are to the Indigenous. The Balinese have big and small ceremonies integrated into their life and even their entire culture. They make rituals multiple times a day, where they create offerings, burn incense, and give thanks to different spirits. Then, they have weekly, monthly, and yearly ceremonies where entire communities or villages honor a Spirit or deity. Also, it was in Bali during a ceremony where I was introduced to the sacred plant medicine cacao, which changed my life.

### *Infusing the Sacred into Our Life*

A ceremony is any intentional space where healing and transformation happen. In a ceremony, we bridge ancient traditions into the present moment. They can be as simple or as elaborate as you'd like them to be—it's all about the intention you have. In a ceremony, we tap into the unseen worlds, accessed through our thoughts, mental images, emotions, bodily sensations, and movement. Oftentimes, ceremony goes hand in hand with a plant medicine, as was shared in Chapter 6. However, anytime you get still and listen, feel what you're feeling, and step into connection with the unseen worlds, you are creating a ceremony.

Sometimes, tears may come; you could sweat or feel fluctuations in your body temperature. You may even witness a miracle and experience magic. In ceremony, we pray, play, and dance, asking for support from our guides, angels, and Ancestors who love us unconditionally. By using our imaginations and remembering our power, we can harness life as a gift, magnetizing more beauty in our lives and in the lives of others. It is equally as important to give yourself the time and space to explore loss, death, or grief. It may seem counterintuitive, but by doing difficult things and acknowledging painful feelings, you will learn how to manifest your best possible life. Through ceremonies, you can fill your life with magic, celebrate the full spectrum of human life, and discover gratitude for both the shadows and the sunshine.

All living humans are descendants of people who have survived catastrophes, pandemics, and traumatic events. Even if it doesn't seem like your life is that bad or you don't feel like there is anything to grieve, if you pause long enough to listen and feel, in the safety of that stillness, something will arise. Furthermore, with access to global news at our fingertips, there is always something happening that could be grieved, from wildfires with suspicious origins, ocean pollution, and the modern-day murder of Indigenous populations, to women being killed in Iran, man-made viruses, and governments overstepping their power for "the greater good." Having access to this much information isn't something our Ancestors had to deal with. It's not your responsibility to be the one to transmute it all. It's actually unhealthy to consume too much information, but know that when you do, your ability to grieve it fully is the only way you'll stay openhearted. We live in a volatile point in the arc of humanity's journey. Through ceremony, we have an opportunity to feel it all, process it, move through it with community, and celebrate life more regularly.

For deep healing to last, it must be done patiently. We do not need any more quick fixes or Band-Aids, like pharmaceutical medications, for what are actually gaping, internal wounds of our soul. Pills, food, alcohol, and entertainment are unsustainable solutions for the deep, nearly unexplainable pains we feel. We need to work within the unseen worlds to find coherence for our body, mind, and soul. Ceremony is what we all need more of to nourish, heal, and restore ourselves. Not only is this simple and what our ancient Ancestors have done for thousands of years, but it is affordable and sustainable.

Reading this book is a ceremony in and of itself because it guides you into a deep connection with your body, mind, and soul, and guides you to reconnect with all things. In a state of presence rather than distraction, you can dance between grief and gratitude, celebrating all of life. Anything and everything can be a ceremony when you are intentional, thoughtful, loving, and feeling into a higher frequency. It is simple yet so profound, for the simplest of things tend to be the most powerful.

### *Shadow Work Is Sacred*

I have so much compassion for us when it seems easier to distract ourselves from painful emotions. There's no shame because we all do it. It's a defining characteristic of humanity, at least at this time of our evolution. That's why I've written this book—to remind you that what you feel is sacred, that you are powerful beyond measure, and that you deserve to live a blissful life, full of gratitude. The journey I went on through the 13 aspects of life, which are now the chapters of this book, took me straight into what I wanted nothing to do with—my shadows.

Sometimes, when I feel like I've done something wrong, it's like I feel bad to my very core. At times, I've felt like a helpless little girl who needs to figure things out so I can feel safe again. I'll try to fix, deny, or pretend that something didn't happen, and as a coping mechanism, I'll distract myself. I am not always okay with the wounded parts of myself that feel ashamed and like I'm not worthy of feeling love. Depending on the intensity of how triggered I am, I'll forget how to hold space for my shadows. But I've learned, by giving myself the time and space to feel and heal, in the safety of that ceremony, I am able to remember my power.

We all have many aspects that create our reality, and our shadows are a natural part of our psyche. Just as past versions of ourselves are full of many positive qualities, we can also hold accumulated childhood hurts, traumas, fears, and anger, until they are acknowledged, loved, and resolved. Similarly, our shadows are our greatest teachers for within their darkness, we find new aspects of light. Take the night sky for example; if it weren't for the ocean of darkness, we wouldn't be able to see the light of the stars. And as you walk upon the ground, if you stand in the sunshine, you will cast a shadow. There is nothing wrong with this, nor is it something to fear or avoid. Your shadows are simply reflections of yourself because of the light shining on you. When you avoid your darkness, your true light is unable to be discovered. Some examples of shadows are holding a grudge, liking it when someone experiences misfortune, or feeling like you must defend yourself even if it means getting angry. These parts may seem like they are "bad," since they're hurtful to ourselves and others. Typically, we feel shameful about what we do that's "wrong," so we feel like those actions, and that we, are unacceptable. But actually, our shadows are an instinctive attempt for us to create safety, regain a sense of control, or ensure we survive a difficult experience.

Take the example of becoming angry while defending yourself. If someone was unintentionally doing something that led you to feel unsafe and like you needed to defend yourself, you may get angry first. Afterward, you may feel guilty and ashamed for reacting. Or if you're like me, you'll feel bad to your core. This is an example of a shadow. The wounded part of yourself is the inner child who felt unsafe, so you needed to defend yourself. When you see it from that perspective, there is nothing "wrong" with what you've done, but you can see how it is hurtful to yourself or others. When you are aware of the "why" underneath any of your actions, it becomes easier to seek resolution, and in so doing, you grow your roots deeper and stronger with those you love.

You have no good reason to fear your own shadows, knowing they naturally come from standing, living in, and being the light. Both the shadows and sunshine create a life that is dynamic, full of texture and variety. If everything was all shadow, we wouldn't be able to see, and if everything was all light, we'd be blinded. When you are standing in the light, it can become intense, and you may turn away and fall back into dark patterns. If you seek out shadows, you may stumble around in the darkness. It's important that you do the work to find balance between the two, so you can grow and be better.

To regain your power is as simple as acknowledging, "Oh, a part of me is feeling unsafe right now. I am feeling angry and like I want this uncomfortable situation to end. I know that reacting is not going to help. Maybe I am not understanding this situation fully. I am first going to create safety within myself by using my breath as a tool to relax my nervous system and stay present in my body, and then I am going to ask the person who I feel unsafe with what their intention of doing that was. And if I continue to feel unsafe, I will remove myself from the situation and come back to it after I am able to be fully present." I'm aware that any normal person would never have this exact dialogue; it's more of a subtle feeling of active surrender that I've given words to. What you may hear is, "Hell no, I gotta go," or "Yeah, I'm not ready for this." Remember to return to your breath, express yourself as best as you can, and trust all will come into the light in its own time.

However, sometimes we do things quickly or intensely without even realizing it. Every time we are triggered and react, this is us being in our shadow; it is simply residual pain from the past being experienced in the present.

This is an opportunity to heal a deep core wound. If you ignore the shadows, you will stay in the darkness of painful emotions. It can be difficult to remember this while experiencing pain we'd rather just ignore. But acknowledging the feelings that come along with the trigger and recognizing what specific wound is being touched on, you can realize what is asking to be seen, held, and felt.

Feeling into your shadows when you're not upset may seem like stirring the pot, yet those feelings are simply energy in motion. They do not define you. By paying attention to passing sensations in the body, thoughts in the mind, and visuals or memories, you will realize you are more than just those sensations. You are the one who experiences the feeling and the one who can witness it. The key to accessing gratitude is not to prefer one thing and suppress another—it's to feel what you feel, see what you see, cry if you need to cry, and remember to laugh with yourself with so much love and not take life too seriously.

Something that has been helpful is to see my shadows as a deer and myself as a jaguar. If you go too quickly, the deer will run, and you won't be able to catch it. If you move thoughtfully and curiously, you will be able to capture it. In capturing it, you can hold, understand, and love it, and then gracefully integrate it.

On the path of healing and awakening, we must release the past so that we can be fully in the present. Only in the present are you able to acknowledge all things, even the difficult experiences that have led you to be right here, right now, reclaiming your power. This is a simple teaching, and sometimes the simplest of things can seem hard to solidify. It gets easier when we are gentle with ourselves and practice being present with what we feel, trusting that our feelings are working for us, not against us. Since this is a lifelong journey, it is important to be gentle and hold yourself tenderly through times of uncovering shadows. And that's exactly what a ceremony is—a place to honor the shadows and the sunshine, grieving when we need to, and embracing gratitude when it comes.

### *Life Is a Ceremony*

For thousands of years, ceremonies have been performed by all cultures to honor and stay connected with our planet's changes, cycles, elements, and many other aspects. Since we come from the planet we live on, we are dynamic beings with primal feelings that also flow through cycles. We are multifaceted, and as long as we have the breath of life in our lungs, we are always evolving and are never just one way during our living days. In the words of Clarissa Pinkola Estés, "Some days I am more wolf than woman, and I am still learning to stop apologizing for my wild."

As shared throughout the book, I have experienced difficulty and pain in life, and I have also caused pain for others. In doing so, I have learned how to do and be better. I always intend on leaving each place better than I found it, yet I am far from perfect. I make big mistakes and even bigger messes. I can be loud, ungracefully honest, rude, and sassy. I can be terrible at communication, and sometimes I mix things up when I speak. Sometimes I communicate better in a language beyond words: the language of feelings, dance, and movement. Sometimes I curse and get angry, yet I'm deeply sensitive and empathetic. I'll cry freely if something or someone touches my heart, and I laugh loudly. We all have "good" and "bad" sides. We are made of shadows and light. We are not just one thing, nor do we ever need to be. We have highs and lows and will experience good and hard times throughout this lifetime. We can flow with what comes and goes, learning to ride the waves so that we do not get swept away or sucked under.

When we embrace our cycles, we can stay in harmony, much like animals and peoples connected to Nature. Every day, we'll experience emotional ups and downs, but when we attune to the cycles of the planet, we'll live with greater balance. If we rise with the sun, with up to 20 minutes of direct sunlight each rising, we signal to our bodies that we are ready for the day, giving our brain the full-spectrum light it needs for balance, energy, and regulation. A lack of sunlight around sunrise and sunset are the top causes of anxiety and depression, something that is a proven fact, but you won't see advertised anywhere. Pharmaceutical companies would quickly be out of business if all of humanity began getting sunlight at dawn and dusk. When the sun falls, the darkness allows for natural melatonin production to work its magic, so we get sleepy and rest fully. During our rest, we have many cycles happening throughout our dream time.

Life itself becomes a sacred ceremony when we live more intentionally. When you live your life with presence, you weave threads of gratitude in the unseen worlds that create beauty in the world around you. By bringing intentionality into our life, we can honor each day as a ceremony. We can also treat every moment as a ceremony by becoming aware of the five things that we are constantly experiencing, which are our thoughts, mental images, emotions, bodily sensations, and movement. These five aspects make up your entire reality. If you want something to change, simply look for where you are having shadowy thoughts, feelings, or mental images. Instead of judging yourself for it, get creative and see how you can shift out of a shadow and into the light of loving awareness.

> *"Rituals are the hands that hold*
> *the community together."*
>
> — Malidoma Patrice Somé

## *Choose Ceremonies That Bring You Life*

Everyone has experienced a form of ceremony with birthdays, holidays, weddings, and other rites of passages. In the United States, our ceremonies revolve around sports, entertainment, music festivals, fashion shows, and other consumer-based gatherings. Each year, the event that brings the most people together in the USA is the Super Bowl. This is a ceremony; however it is one that is directly passed down from the days of gladiators in the Colosseum of Rome. The Roman poet Juvenal coined the phrase "bread and circuses" and with the modern adaptation of "give them bread and circuses and they will never revolt." I know we can collectively do much better and create much more beauty than circus shows, flashing lights, and loud music. I know this because I've experienced the primordial magic of Indigenous ceremonies.

The Aj Q'ijs, or Mayan spiritual guides, practice traditional Mayan fire ceremonies for many reasons. The undertone for every ceremony is to express gratitude and to be in a state of thanksgiving. The ceremonies may be for big life events, celebrations, new beginnings, endings, healing, forgiveness, grieving, letting go, or guidance. Within a fire ceremony, a guide will call in and give thanks to all of the directions, to the Heart of the Earth and the Heart of the Sky, each of the Nawals, and the 13 Mayan numbers—doing this, they're connecting with and expressing gratitude for all aspects of life. All things that are invoked, honored, and revered in a ceremony is a way to give thanks to all things.

There is extensive archaeological evidence that the Maya, and almost all other ancient cultures, would have ceremonies and intentionally consume psychedelic plant medicines. Plant medicine ceremonies can be powerful, deeply transformative, and beautiful experiences. However, as discussed in Chapter 6, you must use discretion. You also must not participate in neo-colonization by going to Central or South America seeking only to get something from these traditions, peoples, and ceremonies. If you, or someone you know goes, you must enter into these lands with an open heart and curious of what you can give. Bring offerings, but ask the locals what they need. Be an ally for them and for future generations.

Being present with everything in your life—the good, bad, messy, the highs and lows, your shadows, and your light—will release fears; heal your body, mind, and soul; and support you in creating a beauty-filled life. When we make space for what we truly want in our lives, we will experience gratitude for all things. This is complete liberation. This is living in bliss.

### *Embodiment Practice: Creating an Altar*

To solidify these teachings and integrate them into your daily life, I recommend creating an altar. This is a sacred space to come to each day; to ground, heal, feel gratitude, and experience life as a ceremony. An altar is a focal point for the sacred. Most Westerners' altar is a TV in the living room, and just like ancient Ancestors, we gather around the fireplace and see, tell, and hear stories. Except nowadays, the fire is in the form of electrical technology and not a crackling bonfire. Therefore, the kind of altar I'm speaking of is one that is less contemporary and more primordial. While there is value in both, and both can connect you to real magic, it's important to have a sacred place you can come to each day centered around intention.

Choose an altar cloth that resonates with you; something colorful, handmade, or perhaps from a parent, grandparent, Indigenous lineage, or spiritual tradition you resonate with. On this cloth, place items that symbolize something special to you. Here you can honor the four directions and the four elements. Place a bowl of water to the south to honor the sacred waters, a candle in the east to honor the fires, a stone or crystal to the west to honor our planet, and a feather in the north to honor the air. You can place a photo of your Ancestors, descendants, or deities that speak to your heart. As often as you can, refresh the altar by replacing the water and adding fresh flowers, new items that come to you, and rearrange the altar whenever you feel called. During the holidays Día de Muertos and Samhain, which fall around Halloween, it's easier to connect with your Ancestors because the veils between worlds are thinner. You can take this opportunity to create an altar to honor those who came before you and prepare the way for those who will come after you.

There is much you can do at an altar. Make it your own, make it sacred, and give yourself at least five minutes at your altar each day. This will help you feel grounded, healthy, balanced during shadowy times, and by becoming present, you'll create a more harmonious life for yourself, no matter what season you're in.

### *Elemental Ceremony*

You can also use a candle to work with all four elements to create a powerful ceremony for yourself or another. The candle wax represents the soil, the flame is fire, the air fans the flame, and the melted wax is liquid, like water. Sit at your altar with your candle in the center. Before you light the fire, create the intention that your prayers or goals will be carried up with the smoke to manifest and become real. As the candle burns, imagine the air being filled with this magic. Maybe your prayer is to call in a new career path, friendship, or a loving relationship. Feel into the qualities you'd like your career, friend, or partner to have and use your imagination to see, feel, and sense them right in front of you.

You can take the ceremony further by drawing them as vividly as you can. It can even be a stick figure because it is about your intention, and then write down what attributes you desire in your best possible life. When you are complete, place it on your altar. Say thank you, or in Maya, maltyox, out loud three times, trusting that what you desire is already on its way to you. Feel grateful as if your intention has already manifested. Leave the drawing on your altar for a time, perhaps a full moon cycle. When you feel ready, bury it, allowing for your intention to be a seed that will sprout and flourish at the perfect time.

CHAPTER 12:

# You Are a Child of Magic

*"Just imagine becoming the way you used to be as a very young child, before you understood the meaning of any word, before opinions took over your mind. The real you is loving, joyful, and free. The real you is just like a flower, just like the wind, just like the ocean, just like the sun."*

— Don Miguel Ruiz

It was the summer of 2010, I was in my early 20s, and I had just gotten the best job of my life. I was hired as a leasing agent at a high-end apartment complex in downtown Los Angeles. Since I was the person getting people to sign papers and hand over the money, the owner of the building took me shopping so I could "look the part." Taking advantage of the situation, I piled up the cart with as many dresses, blouses, and suits that I possibly could.

Even though I didn't remember it at the time, when I was eight, an aunt would take me shopping to get name-brand clothes, which was a big difference from the thrift stores and clearance section of department stores that I was used to. Eventually, she stopped taking me shopping after her and my uncle broke up, instilling a belief within me that being taken care of and given nice things would always come to an end—that any part of my dream life would always just be a taste and wouldn't last.

Therefore, when I was taken dress shopping for my new job, I unconsciously feared this was a limited experience, believing that I better get mine while the getting was good. While I did feel special and taken care of, that magical moment was fleeting. But to the eight-year-old version of myself who was a "good girl" and learned to work hard, I had made it. And to my Mexican American family, I was living a life of their dreams.

I had a good job, I was finding my own way in a big city, and it seemed I was going to make more money than anyone in my family. Everything in my life at the time told me I was in my prime. Not only was that shortsighted, but none of it really mattered to me because underneath the smiles, there was a void that nothing I was experiencing could fill. I was unable to truly be grateful for what I had because even though it looked like I had it all, I felt like I had nothing. I appeared to be an independent woman, I had relative success, and to the unknowing eye, my life looked magical. However, a gnawing emptiness defined my day-to-day life, and the only thing that seemed to satisfy me was the weekend.

On weekends, after grinding through the work week, I would be taken to fancy dinners and the most exclusive clubs in Hollywood. I partied with celebrities, models, businessmen, and professional athletes. For me, the clubs made me feel special. I would sit at a table that not everyone could afford to sit at, with people everyone seemed to want to be with. I could have endless drinks, or take shots of the most expensive tequilas. I would get really excited if our table bought an $800 bottle of champagne so we could shake and pour it all over the dance floor. I laugh at it now, but it was an aimless season in my life. But to be honest, I became addicted to those nights out. They temporarily satisfied the desires of my inner child and gave me access to the most magical life I could find at that time. I've since come to accept and understand why I, and so many others, believe that kind of lifestyle is where we will find happiness. Also, to have gone into and come out of that world means I have a certain level of privilege, which I am aware of and grateful for.

During the week, I was hopped up on caffeine to get me through the 9-to-5 workdays. During the weekend, I numbed my feelings with distraction and masked my pain with consumption, keeping me trapped in cycles of what I thought was a good life. I lived this lifestyle for years, never stopping long enough to ask myself what it was I truly wanted—what my heart desired. Since I was only looking to fill a void, I felt dull, lonely, and disconnected. Deep down, underneath the sparkling lights and bubbly drinks, I knew something wasn't right.

While I now know there is nothing wrong with luxury or glamour, I was using it to brighten up the dullness of my daily life and to feel even a single glimmer of magic. Ultimately, the glitz was a facade. It had no depth, no lasting satisfaction, and was an unsustainable form of escapism. I could look the part in a tight dress on Saturday night, but underneath it all, I still felt like a fearful little girl who would never be enough. Eventually, I learned that clubs and that entire lifestyle only gave me a pseudo sense of magic. For a fleeting moment, you may feel something;

you may mistake an anxious moment of overstimulation as joy, or the watching eyes of many as a sense of being seen and valued. It is exciting on some level, yet it is empty of depth and true connection. That lifestyle perpetuates depression, a sense of separation, and addictions that arise from the need for validation. The glitz and glam comes at a big price, practically in exchange for your soul if you stay there long enough.

Since I hadn't done the work to heal my heart or source my magic and power from within me, I continued to feel unworthy and not good enough. The story I told myself over and over was that the world was a scary place, but if I worked hard, I could have a taste of what I wanted. During my 20s, I took little accountability for my own life and lived within the prison of my own limiting beliefs. Even though I was living a life many think is "making it," deep down I still believed that some people were just lucky. I didn't think I was one of those people because no matter what I did or who I knew, I still felt dull, empty, and lost. For years, I was connected with some of the most famous people in the world, but what I didn't have, and what I really wanted the most, was a connection to myself and the true desires of my inner child.

As is clear, I reached outside myself to search for a more magical life. My life looked fun on the outside, but if you looked close enough, you could see that it was only a mirage. The magic I speak of is not the tricky kind we grew up seeing; that is an illusion. I am speaking of the natural magic our Ancestors and we as children were tapped into. Real magic is felt; it is sustained, it is always accessible, and it is sourced from within us. Reaching outside myself to have a more magical life did help to fill the void I felt inside in the short run, but in the long run it kept me in pain, fear, and suffering.

It was only a few weeks after getting hired as the leasing agent that I was laid off and had to find another job to keep my lifestyle afloat. Throughout my 20s, I hopped from job to job because I found them to be so dull. But in 2014, I moved to Florida with a toxic boyfriend. This decision eventually led me to my lowest point, which ultimately set me on my path to big change. If it wasn't for my "bathroom floor moments," a phrase coined by Elizabeth Gilbert, I may not have discovered the courage to get back up and change my life forever. If I stayed in LA, kept a single job, kept being a "good girl," and kept playing it safe, I may have never discovered the self-trust that comes after ending unhealthy cycles. It's common to end one unhealthy cycle and just get back into another, but when you interrupt the cycles you're in, you give yourself a chance to change—a chance to release one identity for another that is more trusting, more magical, and much more authentic to you.

After reconnecting with my heart, and as I shared in Chapter 6, through the assistance of cacao, I discovered and developed a connection to my inner child. I started to explore what happened to that innocent little girl that made her feel afraid and like she couldn't be her magical self anymore. I found out that my inner child didn't feel safe in the world I was born into and in turn, had created. Instead, she was ignored and denied for years, given quick fixes and only a taste of the magic she yearned for.

Once I began to shed layers of who I wasn't, I could discover who I really was. I realized the fancy and fake life I was living no longer needed to exist. What I really wanted was peace. I wanted connection with myself, to love myself like I had wanted to be loved for so long but ended up being disappointed again and again by family, friends, and lovers. And so my values shifted, and I created a new life for myself—one overflowing with love, magic, playfulness, creativity, and peace. Since I didn't need to pretend or live for anyone else's love, I could give my inner little girl what she always knew she deserved. The more I let my inner child, in all her ages and phases, be heard, the more magical my life became. Understanding my own value and knowing my worth became the catalyst for a wave of creativity and the pathway to abundance. My appreciation for luxury and beauty became a motivation to create and share value with others. By honoring my inner child, I could love myself more, and no parts of myself felt left behind or unsatisfied.

Being your authentic self by connecting to the deep desires of your inner child is critical for you to live a life of peace and true bliss. You will become confident in who you are, and when you love yourself, you find what truly matters. That's what I was looking for all along—the real me. When I began to love myself and not leave my inner child wanting and needing more, I began to receive more love than ever before. I found real sisterhood, incredible communities, and I created a healthy, lasting relationship with Syris. The possibilities are infinite when we open ourselves up to the magic of living authentically.

It's not always going to be easy or be done perfectly. It's probably going to be messy, much like my life has been. By staying connected to your inner wisdom and inner child, any mess you make along the way becomes a chance to rebuild yourself better than you were before. There are many bumps and potential letdowns along the way, to be sure. When every part of you feels seen and acknowledged, when you're no longer chasing something more or avoiding your own pain, you gain a deeper appreciation for what is. When you can honor the mundane and magical, the dull and divine, you can feel grateful for how all of life's experiences have been opportunities for you to learn and grow.

### *What Are Your Gifts?*

Magic is an unseeable force that is always there and available when we listen to the mystery at play in the present. With the gift of our extrasensory perception, we can see, know, or feel the magic with our unique intuitive gifts. Indigenous peoples, like my Mayan Ancestors, knew the power of their magical gifts. Some were seers, prophets, or guides, and others could receive messages in the wind. If someone was blind, deaf, or had a physical disability, they were considered special. In modern times, disabilities greatly disadvantage most people, but to the Indigenous who knew that everything happens for a divine reason, they could realize this was a gift and a calling to tune in to the present. Even the word *disability* means "without ability," but that is only relative to a high-speed, production-driven society. Therefore, Western society needs a fundamental reframe so those of us who experience disabilities can be supported rather than marginalized. Therefore, I've chosen to make a radical choice and see my disability as an opportunity to hone my other senses and receive support, connection, or messages from the unseen realms.

I have tinnitus—a constant ringing—in my right ear. It has never stopped since the day it began. I was in the garden at the home my beloved Syris and I were renting in Guatemala at the height of the pandemic in 2020. I was about to record a podcast when it started. I still got on the call, although I was nervous, a little disoriented, and dizzy. For the first few months, I tried to get rid of it, trying everything from burning ear candles to going to the chiropractor. Understandably, I was attached to my hearing. Being born and raised in unsafe environments, my hearing was something critical for my survival. The fact that the ringing can make me disoriented also contributed to a feeling of not being safe.

Eventually, I was able to grieve the loss of my hearing. But first, I had to recognize that my inner little girl felt she had to stay hypervigilant of her surroundings to be safe. Only after nurturing my inner child, using techniques I'll outline later in this chapter, and fully grieving my losses, was I able to embrace them with genuine gratitude, recognizing them as gifts for my growth and evolution. When I tried to just say I was grateful, then I was only telling myself a lie as a quick fix. Deep within was a sadness for the loss and a feeling of being unsafe. Knowing that seeking this quick fix would only result in disconnection, I went to the only place that would have true answers—within. While I may have lost hearing in one ear, I have gained an ability to listen deeply to my intuition and other metaphysical senses.

To some, this gift would be considered an impediment and is nothing to be grateful for. Tinnitus has driven some people mad, but to the Indigenous, this is a clear sign of a calling. It is common for a healer or shaman to have such gifts. For the Maya, many healers have disabilities or live marching to the beat of their own drum. For example, the midwives that help bring life into this world are chosen for their role through interaction with the unseen realms. Oftentimes, they are gifted with visions, and they learn how to do their important work through communication with certain herbs in the unseen realms, not through any formal education.

We live in a magical world, one where we have the ability to play, dance, and manifest anything we desire to have in our lives. This means we can create both positive and negative things—it's up to us how we use our creative power. As children or adults in a childlike state, we are closest to this remembrance by being tapped into our creativity, imagination, and gifts. When our inner child feels supported, we know that we are worthy of being loved; living this way, we are inherently grateful. However, as is common throughout life as we age, we often experience traumas and tragedies that make us feel unsafe and afraid, seemingly separating us from living in a trusting, playful, and imaginative way.

Do you remember having a vivid imagination? What did you imagine and dream of? How did you play with your magic? Did you ever see anything special or odd? Perhaps you were discouraged from sharing about your "imaginary friends," or maybe like me, you've seen things like angels, fairies, and mystical beings? As a child, I saw what appeared at the time to be an angel in the hallway of my childhood home. But at the tender age of eight or nine, I felt I couldn't tell anyone, or I wouldn't be believed. I never shared what I saw until many years later, after receiving body work on my left shoulder. The memory returned to me, and it gave me a sense of having my own wings, just like what I saw in the hallway. It was a magical experience that I was grateful to have remembered. Some wonder why as humans we so easily forget, and I say it wouldn't feel so good to remember if we hadn't forgotten.

### *Real Magic*

If I had gotten tinnitus 10 years before while working as a leasing agent, I wouldn't have been able to recognize the life-altering change as a gift. I wouldn't have been able to handle nor grieve my hearing loss. It could have been easy to stay in a victimhood mindset rather than choosing to see it from a positive perspective. It wouldn't have connected me to the magic; it would have been just another thing to keep me sad and angry. The ringing is dull, yet if I tune in to it, it sounds like an angelic frequency that goes on forever. In many ways, it is very magical. Now that I've adapted, I usually forget it's happening, but when I listen to it, it feels like a channel has opened me up to the unseen realms.

It came on suddenly and could seem like a handicap. But when closely examined, it's quite a special experience, although I wouldn't have necessarily chosen it for myself. Many gifts happen this way, because your perception of what is, is everything. I chose to let it inspire me and support my life. Yet I do not cling to it as if it must stay. I am fully open to my hearing coming back one day, or not. I accept where I am, I accept this experience as a gift, and I surrender to life's mystery, in full gratitude. And whenever I feel sad, angry, or annoyed at my "disability," it is simply an invitation to grieve what has been or could be, and in its own time, return to accepting what is.

If we don't feel the full spectrum of our feelings, we will create disease from our disabilities. Making the choice to soften and trust in the midst of pain changes everything. Are there any disabilities you have? Maybe yours are more or less involved than mine. Limiting beliefs are self-imposed disabilities. For example, throughout my 20s, my life was defined by thoughts like, *I'm not smart, good, or beautiful enough to have or do what I want.* What stories have you been telling yourself that block you from experiencing the fullness of life? What perspective shifts can you make in your own life to transform something that has caused you pain or turned fear into something that you can be grateful for?

Again, if my onset of tinnitus happened 10 years ago, you would have seen a completely different person. I would not have seen it as a "gift," as I was totally disconnected from my body, mind, and soul. I didn't believe in magic, nor was I connected to my ancestry or Indigenous wisdom teachings. I felt lost, numbed, and I kept myself distracted from my pain by staying busy. If I could just get through my job during the week, then by the weekend I could make something fun happen. In a way, I did create a more magical life, yet that type of magic is unsustainable. It is unsatisfying, unfulfilling, and unhealthy because it is reaching externally to fill the emptiness felt within the heart.

You cannot fill a void in the unseen realms with a physical experience. You must connect with and move within the unseen realms to create sustaining magic in your life. All of the Embodiment Practices in this book are portals to the various aspects of these unseen realms. In this way, you can feel the magic within you and allow the magic to flow forth from there. We are always connected to magic and the unseen worlds, yet we need our practices to remember and hear the wisdom that is there for us. Whenever we do a practice that connects us to magic and expands us into seeing a broader perspective, we give ourselves a chance to feel deep gratitude.

There's real magic and then there's magic that may look real but is actually an illusion. By connecting to your inner child and inner guidance, you will learn to spot the real, and the fake will lose its appeal. The difference between the two is like night and day, yet to those who have forgotten their own magic, like we all do throughout the human experience, we can easily confuse the two. When we remember to source the magic from within, we can find magic within the mundane and in all things. When we give ourselves the time to tune in and listen, we can hone our gifts. By restoring a connection to our fully embodied self: body, mind, and soul, as well as all past versions of ourselves, and especially our inner child, we remember that we will always be a child of magic.

### *Embodiment Practice: Inner Child Healing*

This is a journey to connect with and let your inner child feel safe to be held by you now. Inner child healing can sometimes be difficult, but this is an easy and more playful way to connect. If at any moment you feel overwhelmed, feel your feet resting on the ground. Remember that Mother Nature is always here, able and ready to hold and nurture you, here to help you to feel grounded and safe.

To begin this practice, bring your journal close by; turn on meditation music, healing frequencies, or light shamanic drumming; and close your eyes. If you can, have someone read this journey to you or record yourself reading it. Also, you can read along yourself, pausing to close your eyes and go within.

Lie down or sit up, keeping your spine supported, belly relaxed, jaw relaxed, and your whole body soft. Breathe six times from your nose deep into the belly, and exhale gently through the nose or mouth. Return to normal breathing through your nose.

Use your imagination to see yourself open the front door of your home and enter into a magical garden. See, imagine, feel, or sense yourself moving around this garden. Feel the grass or mud between your toes, the sun warming your face, and a gentle breeze kissing your skin. Now look around at the garden. What do you see? Look at all the different plants. Maybe it looks like a jungle, or maybe it's filled with moss or flowers of your choice. Use your imagination to dream up whatever it is that you'd like to see. Make it fun, playful, and real. Use your imagination to see, sense, taste, hear, and feel gratitude for this beautiful, healing garden. Can you remember yourself as a child and how you could effortlessly use your imagination to transform your experience? Now look around at all the plants and flowers. See if you can imagine or visualize your inner child next to one of your favorite plants. Perhaps you see a big tree. Maybe you see dandelions, sunflowers, or roses. As your adult self, walk toward the child and see the child welcoming you. See the two of you embrace. Does the child tell you anything? Do they ask something? Allow yourself to tell your inner child, "I love you. I am here for you, and I will always be with you to take care of and love you unconditionally. You are safe here. I love you always, in all ways."

Say these words aloud to yourself now: "I love you, I am here for you, and I will always be with you to take care of and love you unconditionally. You are safe here. I love you always, in all ways." Allow the child to lead you somewhere. Play there as long as you like. Then imagine your adult self extending your arms out to your inner child for another hug. This time feel your inner child embrace you and merge within you as a glowing light of joy, innocence, and purity filling you with a sense of wholeness, as you say aloud, "You will always be with me, and I will always keep you safe within me, no matter where we are." Next, imagine and feel your inner child integrated within your adult self. When they're ready to leave, watch them leave the garden together as one.

As you come back into your body and your surroundings, acknowledge that you carry forward the connection to your inner child because you are never truly apart. Notice how your inner child feels secure, knowing they're always loved and protected. Know that this garden is within your heart as well. This is a safe space, and it is accessible to you at any time. Whenever you find yourself desiring to be in a loving and healing space, remember that safety resides within you, and you can use your imagination to tap into it whenever you remember.

CHAPTER 13:

# Bliss Is Your Birthright

*"They say to dance like nobody is watching. I think that implies that we are afraid or ashamed to dance in front of the people. I say dance like everybody is watching. Dance like your children are watching, your Ancestors, your family. Dance for those who are hurting, those who can't dance, those who lost loved ones and those who suffer injustices throughout the world. Let every step be a prayer for humanity. Most of all, dance for the Creator, who breathed into your soul so you may celebrate this gift of life!"*

— Supaman, an Indigenous dancer

We are each here to evolve to a greater state of love. We do this through radically loving ourselves first so that love effortlessly flows out of us. Love is a frequency that comes from nurturing ourselves into a state of gratitude for all our experiences. Every moment provides us a chance to explore the depths of our inner world as well as the vast universe, and make the conscious choice to discover love within it all.

Love is at the core of all human emotions, even those like anger, hatred, envy, or shame. For example, if you notice yourself speaking hesitantly or reacting impulsively, you may find you're feeling insecure underneath your actions. Explore insecurity, and you will find a sense of shame. Explore shame and you will find fear. Look into fear and you will always find a desire to be loved. All emotions that cause suffering come from a desire to be loved. Almost all evil, no matter how extreme, is simply acting out in an attempt to be loved. Every experience is an opportunity to reconnect, reaffirm, reclaim, and deepen into love, if you let it. By doing this, you can live confidently and extend love to everyone—even and especially to those who may be acting out or even working against you—in their own quest for love.

Giving unconditional love is the most powerful state to be in, but it means we must first love ourselves to genuinely give it to others. When we love ourselves, we naturally live in gratitude, reciprocity, and harmony. Then, we can shine authentically and share our expressions of love with the world. It is not always easy to do so, and it must be combined with clear boundaries. It's not always rainbows and butterflies out there, nor should it be. It is a wild, wondrous, complicated, and infinitely complex world. Through it all, we must remember our True Self and truest nature is One with the Source of love, beauty, and bliss, for we are but just a single reflection of this Divinity. As humans, we find it difficult to hold on to this due to feeling separate, different than, or by having traumatic experiences, yet our soul knows this is our truest nature.

We are not meant to be blissed out all the time. We are meant to experience the full range of human emotions because our ability and capacity to feel our depths and pain is a direct reflection with our ability to feel love and joy. In other words, we can't put a limit on our deeper emotions without limiting our higher emotions as well. We must be willing to not have preferences for only feeling good experiences and denying ourselves the opportunity to learn and flourish through the growing pains of difficult ones. We must learn to steady and hold ourselves through the hard times so that we can welcome the good feelings that will come in life. Living means feeling, thus we must feel it all to feel alive. It's a journey to love ourselves through all of it. We must welcome, express, feel, integrate, and accept all parts and sides of ourselves so that we can fully be here now, with open hearts, and exist in the frequency of love.

### *Love Is Your Ultimate Legacy*

Throughout my life, I yearned for something more. I felt this way since childhood, and I didn't really explore this feeling until early last year, around the time this book came through. Sure, I had moments of truth, bliss, and magic, but there were deeper layers of healing that needed to happen to sustainably love myself, reclaim lost parts, and feel wholeness. Intuitively, my heart knew that I was meant for more than what my school, parents, teachers, or society taught me. They taught me to look to an authority outside of myself for the answers. They taught me that my heart, my feelings, and intuition weren't to be trusted. The more I depended or relied on others, the more fragmented, disconnected, and hurt I became.

For most of my life, I struggled with a deep sense of longing and loneliness, and feeling like I didn't truly belong anywhere. What I was searching for, all along, was my True Self. It wasn't until I started to reconnect with my roots and explore the deeper worlds within me that things began to shift. By awakening to my ancestral connection, I not only found the sense of belonging I'd been craving but also discovered that the key to true confidence lies in giving myself permission to be exactly who I am.

Sometimes we need to see something as an example for us to open up to feeling, being, and becoming that which we admire. Life is a Great Mystery, and yet we fit perfectly as a unique piece to the puzzle. Our soul is whole and complete, but it's our human complexities and patterns that cause us to stay in cycles of forgetfulness. When we reclaim our full truth and love our whole self, we can feel complete belonging and acceptance. It is our life's work to remember and put all the pieces of ourselves back together. Throughout the human experience, we will slip up and forget, yet we can always follow the thread of gratitude back to wholeness.

You are an important thread to this Grand Tapestry. You are also the weaver and the weaved. You have free will, yet you're also influenced by mysterious forces of fate, luck, and destiny. You must fully claim your power, wisdom, and sovereignty. Yet you must also remember to soften, surrender, and let Spirit move through you. You are seemingly separate, unique, and one of a kind, which you are! And you're also the same as everyone else, feeling the same shadowy emotions, living with the same feelings of imposter syndrome, lack, overwhelm, and angst. To be human is to be vulnerable to the realities of life. We're constantly caught in these paradoxes, and to make the choice to be conscious, do the work to heal, and live with intention doesn't make everything easier. But it does give you the tools to not get lost in the oceans of suffering, but know that anytime you're feeling resistance, slipping into suffering is a choice.

No one is coming to save you. No one is going to fix you. Because you don't need fixing or saving. What you need is more gentleness, compassion, and curiosity. We all need this from ourselves, yes, but we also need this as a species. Our First Mother needs this for us to continue living on this magical and truly heavenly home. My prayer is that you remember your inherent right to bliss, and may your joy inspire others to join you. Other people may judge you, shame you, or separate themselves from you. For those who do this, all you can hope is that they'll get curious enough to see what's getting in their way from joining you. All you can do is continue right on living the magical life that you're destined to live.

You have so much support, more support than you can imagine. There are no limits to how much you are loved. From your Ancestors, from the plants, your spirit guides, angels, the animals, the elements, and all things above and under the sun. Everything is here for your awakening. Everything can be a catalyst for your continued remembering, as you piece together the mosaic of your own divinity.

This book started by guiding you to the foundational element of any true healing journey—your own body. Now it beckons you to claim the love, bliss, and gratitude that are your birthright to experience within it. The process of tending to all of the 13 aspects of yourself given in the book provides a framework you can keep coming back to. The more you return to these pages, the deeper you will be able to feel, heal, and awaken to who you're meant to be.

Your body isn't just a good place to be—it's the most extraordinary place, for you are a precious and unique embodiment of the Divine. This is cause for continued celebration, as much and as often as you remember the magnitude of this gift. As you integrate the wisdom and reminders contained here, you will transform into a living embodiment of bliss. By connecting with your ancestral roots, recognizing your true essence at a soul level, and loving your full self completely, you will live a life brimming with gratitude. This has been the path of our Ancestors and could very well be the legacy for future generations—only you hold the power to decide.

Love is the legacy you leave. It's how people will remember you. It's how you'll access and become all that you're meant to be. And at the end of your life, it's where you shall return. Leaving a legacy of love means genuinely doing your best, trusting others are doing the same. It's being like water, soft and yet unrelenting. It's being like fire, pure and unchanging while also able to entirely transform. It's being clear and wise like the wind. It's being in right relationship to all things: the planet, the Cosmos, the ones who came before and those that will come after. As Chief Dan George of Tsleil-Waututh Nation said about the legacy we leave, "The time will soon be here when my grandchild will long for the cry of a loon, the flash of a salmon, the whisper of spruce needles, or the screech of an eagle. But he will not make friends with any of these creatures, and when his heart aches with longing, he will curse me. Have I done all to keep the air fresh? Have I cared enough about the water? Have I left the eagle to soar in freedom? Have I done everything I could to earn my grandchild's fondness?"

Remembering your roots, reaching deep into the soils, and stretching high into the sky, you'll awaken your ancestral power and live with gratitude. This is what your Ancestors prayed for you. This is what the Creator has planned for you. Open up to the magic that is this human life, knowing it's okay to forget, it's okay to stumble, because one day, hopefully in this life, or maybe the next, you'll discover all that you are.

### *Embodiment Practice: Dance of Gratitude*

In this practice, you will be expressing gratitude and celebration for this life as a gift. Do this practice somewhere you will feel comfortable to fully express yourself. Stretch before you dance to warm up your body. I like to stretch my neck, my arms, my legs, and warm up the joints, the knees, the ankles, and maybe even shake before dancing.

Put music on a good speaker or headphones so that you can really feel the music, allowing your body to move to the rhythm of the beat. Choose music that will invoke a sense of celebration. To begin, close your eyes, place your hands on your heart. Breathe into your radiant heart. Start to feel or sense deep gratitude for your beating heart—this magnificent organ that has kept you alive through every high and low, and that remains open despite all the challenges you've been through.

Now, with your heart full of gratitude and your body warmed up, let the music guide you. Move in a way that honors your unique spirit, inviting every cell of your being to join in this celebration of life. Remember, this is more than a dance; it's a ritual, a sacred expression of your existence. Let yourself be carried away in the rhythm of the moment, knowing that each step, each beat, each breath is a tribute to the magical gift of being alive. Remember to let go of what you think dance should look like and just move freely to the music. Flow gracefully or erratically. Do whatever you feel like doing to express your gratitude with dance!

When you feel complete after a few songs, bring your hands back to your heart. Close your eyes and breathe here, inhaling in through the nose and exhaling slowly through the mouth. Feel your feet firmly planted on the floor and grounded in the soils, rooting you firmly into your body, knowing that you are safe here, you are free, and you are home.

# Conclusion

Healing happens when we relax into a new reality. We may not have all the words to explain what has happened or what has shifted within us at first, but we will be different, and things will change for the better. In writing the pages of this book, I realized that the act of putting words to paper was itself a journey of transformation—a journey that echoed and brought forth the various chapters of my own life. I journeyed from a place of fear to one of freedom, from feelings of inadequacy to a deeper understanding of my inherent worth. I evolved from feeling lonely to a more profound connection with the essence of my soul. I shifted from feeling uncertain to feeling held and supported by my beloved, my community, my Ancestors, and ultimately, by the Creator. I went from feeling unworthiness to feeling divinely responsible to share my voice so that we can all rise up together. While I still encounter moments of loneliness, grief, and discomfort, these do not define me; instead, they teach me gratitude for the human experience. But each day, I take a step deeper into this wild and wonderful world with my heart wide open.

Remember, genuine transformation is a journey. Life doesn't follow a straight line from hardship to ease; it spirals, revealing deeper layers of our essence. We all bear a shared, sacred responsibility to re-Indigenize our lives by examining and transforming harmful behaviors and unhealthy patterns. In doing so, we reclaim our ancestral wisdom, remember who we are at our roots, and realize what we can become. When we root, we rise. When we are nourished, we blossom.

Our Ancestors want us to live blissfully, surrounded by beauty, and full of gratitude. It's our birthright to reclaim the strength of our forebears, embrace the legacy of our Ancestors, and celebrate the profound wisdom of ancient cultures and traditions. Reclamation and re-Indigenizing can be a challenging and confrontational process. But it doesn't have to stay this way. I've poured my heart out so you can learn from these examples, and I've offered practices to support you on your journey, as they have mine. What I want for you and for all descendants of wise Ancestors is that we live in harmony and live our best lives in gratitude.

Listen not just with your ears, but with your heart, to the wisdom keepers, the children, the elders, the trees, Mother Nature, the Heart of the Sky, and the Heart of the Earth, just like our Ancestors did. Go to Nature to remember your place here. When you fully embrace gratitude for your existence, you will naturally cultivate a life that uplifts both yourself and all that surrounds you.

May you walk in beauty, live in harmony, and find the courage each day to become more deeply connected to your roots.

And so it is.

*Maltyox.*

# Acknowledgments

I am deeply grateful for my Ancestors, those who walked before me, for without them I would not stand where I am today, exactly as I am. It fills me with deep appreciation and honor to be the one chosen to write this book, a tribute to those who preceded me, an offering to those here with me now, and an archive of remembrance for those who come after me. My thanks extend to the Ancestors, the ancient ones, and the elementals, for reassuring me of my belonging, my magic, and my power. To the trees, the waters, the air, the fire—I offer maltyox, deep gratitude, to the good forces that ever remind me that I am loved, seen, held, supported, and appreciated.

I offer immense gratitude to my dear husband, Syris, for his dedication, support, and devotion to the book, and in turn, everything I create. From helping me craft the proposal to clarifying the structure of each chapter, his divine masculine presence provided the foundation this book needed, allowing my creative, feminine energy to flourish and flow.

To my soul sister Sahara, for being one of my biggest advocates, to my big-little sister Priscilla Maya for her unwavering loyalty, Melissa, Davana, Asha, Ana, Christine, Lauren, Emilie, Amber, Heather, Teariki, Marilu, Karen, and so many others, my love is sent to you daily through my eternal gratitude for all you've given me.

To my dear teachers and guides Nana Lu, Nana Maria, Tata Tino, Tata Mark, Tata Izaias, to the trees, the stone people, and to the Wisdom Keepers of Mayan Wisdom, thank you for preserving and passing this wisdom forward for the next generations to carry on. To all of the beautiful beings who have ever joined me in ceremony, the Revival, or the Maltyox Method, in unity I thank you for praying and playing with me.

Thank you to my incredible agent, Steve, who helped me get my dream book published with my dream publishing house. Thus, all my thanks to Hay House Publishing for giving me the space to share my story, uplifting a second-generation immigrant who's moved mountains to be here now, and for helping me build the bridge between Mayan Wisdom and the modern world. To my dear editor, Anna, for seeing the vision and importance of this book, maltyox to you and all the magic you create.

To all descendants of Indigenous peoples who have ever felt stifled, lost, or unsure of themselves, and to the voices who have felt silenced, know that there are many people who would love to support you just as all those I've listed here have supported me. It's my prayer that what's been written in this book provides you with the reminders and nudges to build your most connected, empowered, blissful, and gratitude-filled life.

To my two spirit babies and for my children yet to be born, thank you for blessing me with your loving light and healing cells that will stay with me all my life. Thank you for teaching me, thank you for healing me, and know that you'll never be forgotten.

Finally, thank you to you for being here and for reading this book. May your heart find joy and peace, giving that love to the ones who came before you, those who are with you now, and the ones who will come after you.

# About the Authors

**Christine Olivia Hernandez** is an Aj Q'ij, Mayan Spiritual Guide initiate, and has written many children's books and screenplays. All of her creations are based on her own journey of remembrance, serving as a reminder to reconnect with the innate magic within and around us. She's widely recognized for empowering others from minority communities and Indigenous women's collectives to A-list celebrities—a bridge between Mayan Wisdom and the modern world. Christine has been sharing cacao, her ancestral plant medicine, since 2016 through virtual and in-person programs. She also sells cacao, with direct sources in her ancestral lands of Guatemala and Mexico. This provides work for hundreds of Mayan families, farmers, and women's collectives who process the cacao with traditional methods, and allows buyers to receive organic, fair-trade ceremonial cacao. A facilitator of healing and transformation, she has shared with Poosh Wellness, Alo Yoga, Yoga Journal, notable masterminds, and thousands of people worldwide. With all she does, Christine inspires others to tap into their magic and live with gratitude. Find out more at **iamchristineolivia.com**.

**Syris Elijah King-Klem** is a cross-genre author, writer, and editor. Specializing in memoirs, business/leadership, and spirituality, he has guided over 10 authors to traditionally publish their books and assisted many more with self-publishing. An Air Force veteran, Syris has devoted his life to the craft of storytelling, knowing that through the stories we tell, we can shift, determine, and create our reality. He's also an actor, screenplay writer, and film producer living in Los Angeles, CA. Find out more and connect directly with him at **syriskingklem.com**.

## Hay House Titles of Related Interest

*YOU CAN HEAL YOUR LIFE, the movie*
starring Louise Hay & Friends
(available as an online streaming video)
www.hayhouse.com/louise-movie

*THE SHIFT, the movie,*
starring Dr. Wayne W. Dyer
(available as an online streaming video)
www.hayhouse.com/the-shift-movie

***

*YOU ARE THE MEDICINE: 13 Moons of Indigenous Wisdom, Ancestral Connection, and Animal Spirit Guidance* by Asha Frost

*SPIRIT TALKER: Indigenous Stories and Teachings from a Mi'kmaq Psychic Medium* by Shawn Leonard

*THE EARTHCRAFT ORACLE: A 44-Card Deck and Guidebook of Sacred Healing* by Juliet Diaz and Lorraine Anderson

*WISDOM DEL ALMA: 44 Affirmation Cards to Activate Your Inner Diosa* by Christine Gutierrez

All of the above are available at your local bookstore
or may be ordered by visiting:

Hay House India: www.hayhouse.co.in
Hay House USA: www.hayhouse.com®
Hay House Australia: www.hayhouse.com.au
Hay House UK: www.hayhouse.co.uk

All of the above are available at your local bookstore,
or may be ordered by contacting Hay House (see next page).

***

We hope you enjoyed this Hay House book. If you'd like to receive our online catalog featuring additional information on Hay House books and products, or if you'd like to find out more about the Hay Foundation, please contact:


HAY HOUSE

**Hay House Publishers (India) Pvt Ltd**
Muskaan Complex, Plot No. 3,
B-2, Vasant Kunj, New Delhi 110 070
Phone: +91 11 41761620
www.hayhouse.co.in

—

***Published in the United States by:***
Hay House LLC, P.O. Box 5100, Carlsbad, CA 92018-5100
(760) 31-7695 or (800) 654-5126
www.hayhouse.com® • www.hayfoundation.org

***Published in Australia by:***
Hay House Australia Publishing Pty Ltd
18/36 Ralph St., Alexandria NSW 2015
*Phone:* +61 (02) 9669 4299
www.hayhouse.com.au

***Published in the United Kingdom by:***
Hay House UK Ltd
1st Floor, Crawford Corner,
91–93 Baker Street, London W1U 6QQ
*Phone:* +44 (0)20 3927 7290
www.hayhouse.co.uk


—


**Let Your Soul Grow**

Experience life-changing transformation—one video at a time—with guidance from the world's leading experts.

www.healyourlifeplus.com

# Free e-newsletters from Hay House, the Ultimate Resource for Inspiration

Be the first to know about Hay House's free downloads, special offers, giveaways, contests, and more!

Get exclusive excerpts from our latest releases and videos from ***Hay House Present Moments.***

Our ***Digital Products Newsletter*** is the perfect way to stay up-to-date on our latest discounted eBooks, featured mobile apps, and Live Online and On Demand events.

Learn with real benefits! ***HayHouseU.com*** is your source for the most innovative online courses from the world's leading personal growth experts. Be the first to know about new online courses and to receive exclusive discounts.

Enjoy uplifting personal stories, how-to articles, and healing advice, along with videos and empowering quotes, within ***Heal Your Life.***

**Sign Up Now!**

***Get inspired, educate yourself, get a complimentary gift, and share the wisdom!***

**Visit www.hayhouse.com/newsletters to sign up today!**

HAY HOUSE

HAYHOUSE online learning

# MEDITATE. VISUALIZE. LEARN.

*Get the* **Empower *You***
Unlimited Audio *Mobile App*

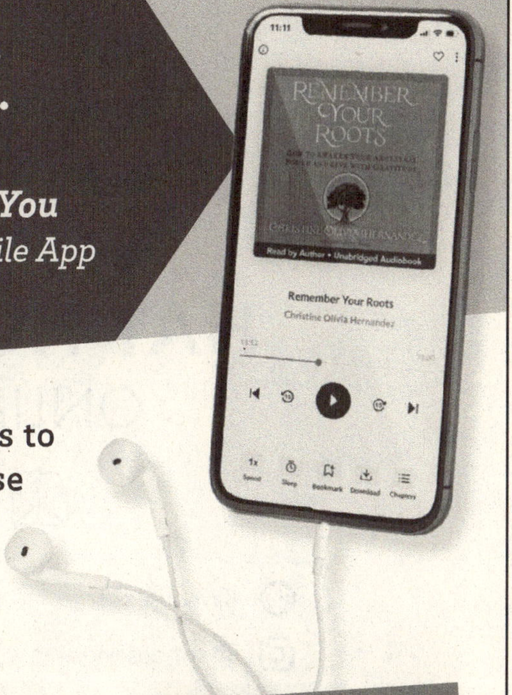


## Get unlimited access to the entire Hay House audio library!

**You'll get:**

- 500+ inspiring and life-changing **audiobooks**
- 700+ ad-free **guided meditations** for sleep, healing, relaxation, spiritual connection, and more
- Hundreds of audios **under 20 minutes** to easily fit into your day
- **Exclusive content** *only* for subscribers
- **New audios** added every week
- No credits, **no limits**

**Listen to the audio version of this book for FREE!**

"★★★★★ **I ADORE this app.** I use it almost every day. Such a blessing. – Aya Lucy Rose"

Scan me with your phone camera!

HAY HOUSE

# TRY FOR FREE!

Go to: hayhouse.com/listen-free

HAY HOUSE

CONNECT WITH

# HAY HOUSE

ONLINE

hayhouse.co.in

@hayhouseindia

@hayhouseindia

@hayhouseindia

Join the conversation about latest products, events, exclusive offers, contests, giveaways and more.

*'The gateways to wisdom and knowledge are always open.'*

**Louise Hay**